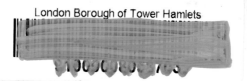
The Author

Rosemary Conley is the UK's most successful diet and fitness expert. Her diet and fitness books, videos and DVDs have consistently topped the bestseller lists with combined sales in excess of nine million copies.

Rosemary has also presented more than 400 cookery programmes on television and has hosted several of her own TV series including *Slim to Win with Rosemary Conley*, which was broadcast in ITV Central and Thames Valley regions in 2007.

In 1999 Rosemary was made a Deputy Lieutenant of Leicestershire. In 2001 she was given the Freedom of the City of Leicester, and in 2004 she was awarded a CBE in the Queen's New Year Honours List for 'services to the fitness and diet industries'.

Together with her husband, Mike Rimmington, Rosemary runs four companies: Rosemary Conley Diet and Fitness Clubs, which operates an award-winning national network of almost 200 franchises running more than 2000 classes weekly; Quorn House Publishing Ltd, which publishes *Rosemary Conley Diet & Fitness* magazine; Rosemary Conley Licences Ltd; and Rosemary Conley Enterprises.

Rosemary has a daughter, Dawn, from her first marriage. Rosemary, Mike and Dawn are all committed Christians.

Also in Arrow by Rosemary Conley

Rosemary Conley's
Gi Hip & Thigh Diet

The fastest, healthiest weight and inch loss plan – ever!

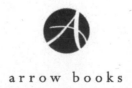

arrow books

Published in the United Kingdom by Arrow Books in 2008

15

Copyright © Rosemary Conley Enterprises 2008

Rosemary Conley has asserted her right under the Copyright, Designs and Patents Act 1988 to be identified as the author of this work

Arrow Books
Random House Group Limited
20 Vauxhall Bridge Road, London SW1V 2SA

www.rbooks.co.uk

Addresses for companies within The Random House Group Limited can be found at: www.randomhouse.co.uk/offices.htm

The Random House Group Limited Reg. No. 954009

A CIP catalogue record for this book is available from the British Library

ISBN 9780099517771

The Random House Group Limited makes every effort to ensure that papers used in its books are made from trees that have been legally sourced from well-managed and credibly certified forests. Our paper procurement policy can be found at: www.randomhouse.co.uk/paper.htm

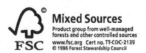

Mixed Sources
Product group from well-managed forests and other controlled sources
www.fsc.org   Cert no. TT-COC-2139
© 1996 Forest Stewardship Council

Edited by Jan Bowmer
Designed by Roger Walker

Typeset in FS Albert

Printed and bound in Great Britain by Clays Ltd, Elcograf S.p.A.

Acknowledgements

I have enjoyed writing this book for many reasons. It has been exciting to relive some of the wonderful memories of writing my original Hip and Thigh Diet more than 20 years ago. Then, more recently, I had the challenge of upgrading and rewriting it to include my very latest and proven philosophy of incorporating low-Gi foods into low-fat, calorie-controlled meals and combining this with regular exercise to give the healthiest and fastest weight and inch losses ever!

I could not have written this book without the help and support of the great team with whom I have the pleasure of working, so thank you to chef Dean Simpole-Clarke, who has created lots of delicious recipes for you to enjoy; to my secretary Anja Zeman for calculating the nutrition content of the meals; to my good friend and colleague Mary Morris, fitness expert, for her encouragement and help in putting together the exercise chapters; to Teresa Keates for following the diet religiously for four weeks – she lost 14lb! – and for testing the shopping lists for me.

The introduction of Portion Pots in this diet involved a lot of work in establishing portion sizes and the corresponding weights and calorie calculations. My daughter, Dawn, undertook this meticulous task on my behalf. Without her help I do not see how this book could have been made so helpful and comprehensive for the dieter. Thank you, Dawn, for your tremendous input, hard work and perseverance.

Thank you also to my husband, Mike, for his love and support not only during the writing of my original Hip and Thigh Diet, but throughout the preparation of all my subsequent diets, including this one.

As always, I want to thank my very hard-working editor, Jan Bowmer, who magically pulls together my somewhat disjointed manuscript into a readable volume! Also, thanks to Roger Walker for designing the inside pages and to my commissioning editor, Hannah Black, at Random House for her support and belief in yet another diet book from me! And to everyone else who has played a part in making this book what it is. Thank you all.

Useful information

Body weight conversions

Pound (lb)	Stone (st)	Kilogram (kg)	Pound (lb)	Stone (st)	Kilogram (kg)
1		0.5	9		4.1
2		1	10		4.5
3		1.4	11		5
4		1.8	12		5.4
5		2.3	13		5.9
6		2.7	14	1	6.3
7	½	3.2	28	2	12.7
8		3.6			

Linear measurements

Inch (in)	Feet (ft)	Millimetre (mm)	Centimetre (cm)
⅛		3	
¼		5	
½			2.5
1½			4
2			5
2½			6
3			7.5
3½			9
4			10
5			13
6			15
7			18
8			20
9			23
10			25
12	1		30

Spoon measures

1 teaspoon (tsp) = 5ml   1 tablespoon (tbsp) = 15ml

Abbreviations and symbols used

lb	pound	mm	millimetre
g	gram	cm	centimetre
kg	kilogram	kcal	calorie
st	stone	tsp	teaspoon
ml	millilitre	tbsp	tablespoon
in	inch	Ⓥ	suitable for vegetarians
ft	foot	❄	suitable for home freezing

Contents

The diet in this book is based on sound healthy eating principles. However, it is important that you check with your doctor or GP before following any weight-reducing plan. Diabetics should always follow the eating guidelines recommended by their GP or medical practitioner.

The Hip & Thigh Diet Phenomenon

Would you like to get rid of your excess pounds fast, easily and safely and still eat lots of delicious foods? Well, now you can! You won't believe how quickly you can lose weight on my Gi Hip and Thigh Diet! You could shed 7lb in the first two weeks and then progress to the very easy-to-follow Phase 2 of the diet until you reach your ultimate goal.

The diet is extremely flexible as all the menus are interchangeable. You can select which breakfast, lunch or dinner you like best for each day – and there are loads to choose from. All the calorie counting has been done for you to make it even easier and more effective and there's no need to count fat grams or Gi values. Also, you can tone up as you slim down with an easy-to-fit-into-your-life daily activity challenge. Losing weight has never been simpler, faster, healthier or more fun!

How it all began

My original *Hip and Thigh Diet* was published in 1988 after I discovered, quite by accident, the dramatic effect of eating a diet that was very low in fat.

It all started in 1986 when I was diagnosed with a gall-stone problem after falling ill and being rushed into hospital. The doctors recommended immediate surgery to remove my gall bladder. As I was in the process of winding up a slimming club I had been running for an international magazine company, I couldn't afford the eight weeks off to recover from, what was then, a major operation. I was told that the only alternative was to eat a very-low-fat diet and then, maybe, I would be all right. So that's what I did, and then a miracle happened. I lost 6lb of fat – that's 2.7 kilos – and it all seemed to go from my hips and thighs!

I had suffered with fat, horrible thighs since my teens. In my efforts to reduce the ugly cellulite that was so prevalent I even used to massage them with a rolling pin! At my heaviest I weighed 10st 4lb, which was a lot for my small-framed, 5ft 2in body, and when I started on the very-low-fat diet, I weighed 8st 6lb. It took six weeks to lose that 6lb and for the first time in my adult life I had slim thighs!

Members of the exercise classes I was teaching at the time couldn't help noticing my changing shape and begged me to design a very-low-fat diet for them. This I gladly did and when they, too, started losing inches from their hips and thighs, I realised I had hit on something significant.

I'd already had three books published, and this was my opportunity to write a fourth. First, I needed to test the diet further, so I enlisted the help of local radio to ask for volunteers to follow the diet for eight weeks and then fill in a questionnaire. The requests flooded in.

Eight weeks later, the completed questionnaires began to arrive. The results were astounding. Everyone who sent them back had lost weight, but what surprised members of the trial team most was the reduction in inches – particularly from around their hips and thighs. They had written comments such as, 'I have tried more diets than I care to remember but none has had the effect of slimming down my enormous thighs as much as your diet. I couldn't be more thrilled – or grateful!'

So I analysed the results of the trial dieters and collated their encouraging comments and inspiring reports of health benefits. I extended the diet from the small version I had supplied to my trialists and, some months later, the book was ready to send off to the publishers. I had a feeling it was going to be a bestseller.

I was keen to have the book serialised in a national newspaper. A friend and ex-colleague, Christine, spoke to a contact of hers at the *Sunday Express* and asked them to listen to what I had to say about the diet. They did, a deal was made and the serialisation ran over the first two weeks of January 1988 to coincide with publication of the book.

After Christmas, people are ready to follow a diet and my *Hip and Thigh Diet* seemed to work brilliantly for those who tried it. The book shot to No. 2 in the bestseller charts and by the following week it was No. 1. It stayed in that coveted position for many months. The book 'flew' off the shelves and was reprinted no less than nine times that year.

I started to receive a huge postbag of letters from people who were following the diet and achieving amazing success. My husband, Mike, and I worked from a little office at home, coping with our vast mailbag and fending off the press, who all wanted to interview me. Soon videos and TV offers followed and by August 1988 we were off to Australia on book tour where the *Hip and Thigh Diet* became a No. 1 bestseller, too.

It became obvious that people wanted more, so I wrote a

sequel and my *Complete Hip and Thigh Diet* was published in 1989. By now we had a couple of staff in our office – first Diane, then Angie – to cope with the workload, both of whom still work with us today.

My *Complete Hip and Thigh Diet* shot straight to No. 1 in the UK bestseller charts and, later, also in Australia, New Zealand, Canada and South Africa. It went on to sell a monumental two million copies and was reprinted 25 times! Little did I know that my *Hip and Thigh Diet* books would provide the foundation for the low-fat eating trend we know so well today.

Why was my Hip and Thigh Diet so successful?

The diet's success was due to its low-fat eating formula. There's no doubt that the fat we eat is stored as fat on our bodies. Research has shown that fat is at the bottom of the priority table when the body calls upon its food stores for energy. Only when its supplies of protein and carbohydrate have been exhausted will it draw on its fat stores for fuel. On a calorie-controlled low-fat diet, such as the one in this book, you won't replenish those fat stores, so you lose lots of inches. That's why my hips and thighs slimmed down so dramatically, because it's where I stored most of my fat. After I dramatically reduced my fat intake, those stores became smaller and I literally shrank. It is as simple as that.

Moreover, my Hip and Thigh Diet was very easy to follow – dieters could eat any food they liked as long as it was low in fat, and they could have unlimited portions of rice, pasta, potatoes and vegetables, providing they did not add any fat during cooking or serving. They were allowed three meals a day and could drink alcohol in moderation. There were no calories to count and everyone loved the freedom of choice.

However, over time, followers of the diet found that their rate of weight loss slowed down and this was down to the fact that their servings of rice, pasta and potatoes had become larger! I therefore modified the diet to make it more prescriptive, specifying portion sizes and recommending a daily exercise routine in my subsequent book, *Inch Loss Plan*, which was published in 1990. This, too, became a No. 1 bestseller and went on to sell over 800,000 copies. People liked the fact that each day they were told exactly what to eat and which exercises to do.

Further books followed – almost 30 in fact – along with as many fitness videos, now available as DVDs, and a national TV series. In 1993 we launched Rosemary Conley Diet and Fitness Clubs as a franchise and, in 1996, *Rosemary Conley Diet & Fitness* magazine. It has been an incredibly exciting journey and I have enjoyed every moment.

A new decade, a new diet

During the 20 years between publication of my first *Hip and Thigh Diet* and this *Gi Hip and Thigh Diet* the number of low-fat food products available in UK supermarkets has gone from just a few low-fat or lower-fat alternatives to tens of thousands of options. There are now endless food ranges to choose from where 'low fat' is the key selling point.

Confronted by so much choice, we can no longer rely on eating low-fat foods alone if we want to lose weight; we have to consider our calorie intake as well. Also, it became apparent in the late nineties that people who couldn't live without eating the occasional bar of chocolate or bag of crisps felt they weren't able to go on my low-fat diet. With that in mind, I have modified the eating plans over the last few years to allow slimmers to enjoy a few high-fat treats if they so choose.

To ensure an optimal level of weight loss, I recommended that each individual stick to a daily calorie allowance based on their basal metabolic rate (BMR), which is scientifically calculated according to their gender, age and current weight. Then, adding in some exercise would dramatically accelerate their rate of weight loss so that they could eat plenty yet still lose weight. And it worked brilliantly.

The Glycaemic Index

Then came the Glycaemic Index (Gi), which was originally created to help diabetics. It was discovered that eating certain carbohydrate foods which caused their blood sugar to rise slowly helped stabilise their insulin levels. Not only that, but it soon became evident that eating low-Gi foods also improved heart health.

But there is another big bonus that comes from eating a low-Gi diet. As low-Gi foods are less processed and higher in fibre than other carbohydrates, they take longer to digest and therefore keep us feeling fuller for longer. Just what the dieter needs – a diet that fills them up and prevents hunger pangs between meals!

A great deal of work has now been done to establish which foods have a low Glycaemic Index rating, but it isn't an exact science. Ratings can be manipulated by increasing other elements, such as fat, during the food manufacturing process and, as a result, some high-fat foods have been labelled as 'low Gi'.

So, take the trouble to check the nutrition labels of food products, as eating high-fat foods will not help you to lose weight.

For simplicity, I prefer not to state the calculated Gi values in my diets. I select carbohydrate foods that are known to have a low-Gi ranking and that are also low in fat. This makes the diet really healthy. I eat this type of diet every day and I certainly feel better for it and find I can easily maintain my weight.

So here I am celebrating 20 years of the Hip and Thigh Diet and putting together a twenty-first century version for a whole new generation of readers. Over the last couple of decades, I have been privileged to work with some top nutrition scientists and fitness experts from whom I have learned so much. I certainly know a great deal more now than I did in 1988 – and it's all in this book!

2

The New Gi Hip and Thigh Diet – How It Works

This Gi Hip and Thigh Diet is based on a culmination of two extensive trials and my own experience over the years. I have also borne in mind the desires and needs of the dieter who wants to lose weight fast.

Perfect portion control

Overestimating portion sizes is the biggest single reason why dieters don't lose weight as fast as they think they deserve to. It's easy to become complacent and that's when the extra calories can creep in and slow down your weight-loss progress. Portion control therefore is crucial to successful weight loss.

However, it is unrealistic to imagine that we are going to weigh our portions of rice or pasta on the scales every time we want to eat them. That's why I have created my Rosemary Conley Portion Pots. These are handy tools for measuring cereal, rice, pasta and other basic foods.

The pots come in four different colours and sizes with the following liquid capacities:

blue	80ml
yellow	125ml
red	250ml
green	330ml

When measuring solids, the quantities and weights in the portion pots will vary according to the density of the specific food (see pages 285–7). But you don't have to worry, as I have done all the relevant calculations for you in this Gi Hip and Thigh Diet. The pots also come with an easy guide as to which pot holds how much of various everyday foods. They make it incredibly quick and simple to accurately gauge your portion sizes that it will soon become automatic. So, if you stick to the recommended menus in this diet and make sure you eat the correct quantities of foods, you will maximise your weight-loss progress.

My portion pots are such a great aid that I have two sets and, for speed and convenience, I keep the appropriately sized pot in the relevant food storage container. For instance, I keep the yellow one with my muesli and I know that just one scoop is 183 calories-worth, and I keep a blue one with my porridge oats (one scoop of dry oats is equivalent to 125 calories). A blue portion pot of *uncooked* basmati rice will give me 205 calories when cooked, the same as a red portion pot of *cooked* basmati rice. (For details of how to order the pots, see the back of this book.)

The optimum weight- and inch-loss formula

I believe that I now have the optimum formula to effect a quick weight and inch loss, one that combines a healthy, nutritious eating plan with a fitness regime that will burn fat, strengthen your muscles and, as a result, increase your fitness and fat-burning potential not only now but also well into the future. I'll explain exactly how this happens in a later chapter.

This diet and fitness programme is designed in such a way that you will experience a significant weight loss in the first two weeks as you follow Phase 1, the Fat Attack Fortnight. Then, having lost around 7lb in the first 14 days and seen a significant number of inches disappear from around your waist, hips and thighs, you will hopefully feel totally committed to continue on the more generous Phase 2 of the Gi Hip and Thigh Diet.

There is a choice of a set diet plan to follow or you can plan your own daily menus from the meal options given in chapter 11. Remember, all the meals are totally interchangeable, so if there is one breakfast you particularly like, you can have it every day if you wish. There is also a daily exercise challenge to speed up your weight loss and tone you up as you slim down.

After the first two weeks, you may also add a daily treat, which can be high or low fat and high or low Gi, plus you can enjoy an alcoholic drink if you want to. In addition, if your personal calorie allowance permits, you can include a dessert each day to have with your evening meal or you can increase your portion sizes of foods such as cereal, rice, pasta and potatoes. Again, all this has been calculated for you, using the portion pots.

This diet is incredibly versatile. You can choose which meals you want to eat from the vast number of options and you can eat them when you want. You can eat or drink your treats whenever you choose or save them up for a special occasion. Also, you can use your daily milk allowance of 450ml/¾ pint in tea and coffee and on your breakfast cereals. If you don't drink much milk, you can swap 150ml milk for 1 × 125ml low-fat yogurt with a maximum of 75 calories.

This diet is easy to fit into your lifestyle and you won't feel you are on a diet at all – it will just become a new way of eating.

I have also included lots of delicious recipes for you to try and I promise you that your family will love them, too. They have been created by chef Dean Simpole-Clarke, who has worked with me on television as well as on my books and my *Diet & Fitness* magazine for the last ten years.

Once you are on Phase 2 of the diet, if at any time you want to give your weight-loss progress a boost, just select your meals as stated and miss off the treat, puddings and alcohol. Don't be tempted to do this too regularly, though, as it could slow down your metabolic rate and delay your success in the longer term.

If you get into the habit of using the portion pots whenever you are serving your cereal, rice, pasta and other foods, you will speed up your weight loss like a dream.

When you have lost all your unwanted weight you will be able to maintain it by following the principles of the eating habits you have learned. You won't need to follow the calorie-counted meal options but you will automatically find yourself selecting low-fat foods as your taste buds will have changed. I am sure you will find that high-fat foods won't taste as good any more. Also, once you've achieved a fabulous figure, you will find yourself deciding that you'd rather have a slim body than a cream cake!

I guarantee that if you follow this diet it will work. You will feel so much healthier and more confident – like a brand new person in a sensational, new and fitter body. So, enjoy the journey.

3

A Quick Guide to Gi

Gi stands for Glycaemic Index, which ranks foods according to the speed at which they are digested and absorbed into the bloodstream. As mentioned earlier, it was originally created to help diabetics stabilise their insulin levels, but it has now been scientifically proven to be a healthy way of eating for everyone. And making low-Gi choices needn't be difficult.

In the 36 years I have been writing diet plans, I have never witnessed such incredible successes as I did after my first low-Gi diet book, the *Gi Jeans Diet*, was published in 2006. This new *Gi Hip and Thigh Diet* book builds on those successes and is devoted to helping YOU achieve and enjoy amazing results, too.

How does Gi aid weight loss?

We all know now that to lose weight fast and healthily we have to consume a balanced, healthy, low-fat diet and eat fewer calories than our bodies use so that we call on our fat stores to make up the shortfall. We then need to spend more calories by being more active and doing more exercise to speed up the weight-loss process.

So where does Gi come in? As well as being good for our health, low-Gi foods keep us feeling fuller for longer, thus reducing hunger pangs and cravings. This is the very best news if you are on a weight-reducing plan as you won't go hungry on this Gi Hip and Thigh diet even though you are likely to be consuming fewer calories than you are used to eating.

Which foods are low Gi?

The Glycaemic Index relates primarily to carbohydrates — that's bread, pasta, rice, potatoes and cereal. Here is a quick guide to selecting low Gi options:

Bread Choose natural, stoneground or wholegrain brown bread with bits of grain in it instead of white or highly processed brown. Wholemeal bread is often processed too and therefore has quite a high Gi ranking.

Pasta All pasta is low Gi. Eat it with low-fat, tomato-based sauces in preference to creamy ones (unless they are low fat) while you are trying to lose weight.

Rice Basmati rice has a lower Gi than most other types. Brown rice is also considered low Gi, although it takes longer to cook.

Potatoes Have sweet potatoes in preference to old ones. They can be cooked in exactly the same way — you can boil then mash them or bake in the oven in their skins and serve with a healthy topping such as baked beans or cottage cheese. Also try dry-roasting them. Just peel them and par-boil for 5 minutes and then just place them on a non-stick baking tray on the top shelf of your oven and cook for 40 minutes. Without any added fat they will still go brown round the edges just like old potatoes. They taste fabulous and children love them, too. Waxy new potatoes are also low Gi. Cook and eat them with their skins still intact for extra fibre.

Cereals Go for unprocessed cereals such as oat-based varieties, including muesli, or any cereal that is natural and high in fibre, like All-Bran, Shredded Wheat, Weetabix, bran flakes, porridge oats, and so on. Special K is also low Gi.

Does low Gi mean low fat?

No. Adding fat to food products can reduce its Gi rating, and some manufacturers do this so that they can advertise their products as low Gi. When you are trying to lose weight, this, of course, defeats the object! So always look for low-fat foods (with 5% or less fat) and ingredients and try to find low-Gi ones, too, whenever possible.

Does everything I eat have to be low Gi?

Not at all. By making a few simple changes as suggested above you can turn your normal low-fat diet into a mostly low Gi one, but you can still have higher Gi treats occasionally to satisfy your taste buds. After you have completed the Fat Attack Fortnight, you will be allowed a 100-calorie treat each day and this can be high fat and high Gi if you wish. You can also save up your treats over seven days for a bigger treat or special occasion.

Should I continue to eat low Gi in the future?

For the good of your general health, yes. Most of the original trial dieters who followed my first low-Gi diet said that they enjoyed making these changes to their diet and were really happy to carry on this new way of eating after losing their excess weight. The biggest benefits were that they felt much healthier and that the food they ate filled them up so that they didn't feel hungry.

So, if you want to lose weight, look and feel ten years younger and have bags more energy, you will find all the information you need in this book. This diet really does work!

Gi at a glance

* Choose high-fibre or oat-based cereals for breakfast rather than highly refined ones.

* Select wholegrain or stoneground bread or loaves containing seeds and grains.

* Basmati rice has a lower Gi than other varieties.

* Sweet potatoes and waxy, new potatoes have a lower Gi than old potatoes. Cook them with their skins intact for extra fibre.

* Pasta is a good low-Gi option.

* Add beans and pulses to stews and casseroles, salads and soups to add bulk and reduce the overall Gi rating of your meal.

* Eat fruit in place of cakes and biscuits.

* Choose bananas that are slightly under-ripe as they have a lower Gi rating than over-ripe ones.

* Drink water in place of high-sugar drinks.

4

Why Do You Want to Lose Weight?

There are many benefits to losing your excess weight. You will shed lots of fat from your body, making it easier to move about, more comfortable to lie down in bed, sit in a chair, bend down, reach up or even just walk without difficulty or getting tired so easily. Your thighs won't chafe together, your waist-band won't 'cut' you in half, you won't get so out of breath and you'll sleep much better.

Once you are slim, you will no longer feel self-conscious and you won't have to rely on buying clothes only in outsize shops. People will start noticing you and treating you with respect. As one dieter told me, 'People used to talk about me but now they talk *to* me.'

Isn't all that worth making some simple changes to your lifestyle and putting in a little effort? And I haven't even mentioned the improvements to your health and looks, such as lower cholesterol and blood pressure, better digestion, easing of joints, less back pain, younger-looking, clearer skin, brighter eyes, stronger nails and shinier hair.

Reasons for Losing Weight

Before you start the diet, think about *why* you want to lose weight so that you can get your thoughts in order and are truly ready to embark on a journey that is going to transform your body and your health.

If you have a specific goal to aim for, you are much more likely to achieve your weight-loss target. So take time to acknowledge your reasons for wanting to be slim. Maybe you lack self-confidence, or your clothes are too tight and uncomfortable? Or is it because you hate looking at yourself in the mirror at the moment? Perhaps you feel tired all the time and are concerned about your health? Tick the relevant boxes on pages 20–21 and add some more of your own.

Now realise how those feelings will be reversed when you reach your goal weight. You'll start to stand up for yourself and you will be so much happier. Your self-confidence will rocket, you'll adore shopping for clothes because everything you try on will fit in all the right places, you will love looking in the mirror, going out, dressing up. Your health will be transformed and you will feel much younger.

How much weight will I lose?

If you stick rigidly to the diet, don't cheat and exercise every day, you can lose 2–3lb a week, even more if you are very overweight. Where people often go wrong is that, after the first couple of weeks, they start guessing their portion sizes and end up eating more than they realise, which can slow down their progress. That's why I recommend you use my portion pots (see pages 285–7) to help you to stay right on track.

I want to lose weight because:

- ☐ I WANT TO BE HEALTHIER

- ☐ I WOULD LIKE TO WEAR SIZE ___ CLOTHES

- ☐ I WANT TO STOP FEELING EXHAUSTED

- ☐ I WANT TO FEEL FITTER

- ☐ I WANT TO FEEL HAPPIER WITH MYSELF

- ☐ I WANT TO BE MORE SELF-CONFIDENT

- ☐ I WANT TO LOOK YOUNGER

- ☐ I WANT TO BE ABLE TO JOIN IN WITH SPORTS AND ACTIVITIES

- ☐ I WANT TO BE ABLE TO JOIN IN ACTIVITIES WITH MY CHILDREN/FAMILY

- [ ] I WANT TO HAVE MORE ENERGY

- [ ] I WANT TO SLEEP BETTER

- [ ] I WANT TO LIVE LONGER

- [ ] I WANT TO HAVE A LIFE

- [ ]

- [ ]

- [ ]

- [ ]

- [ ]

- [ ]

- [ ]

- [ ]

- [ ]

- [ ]

Get Ready

The week before you begin the diet, start making your preparations. Clear your fridge and cupboards of foods you will no longer need to eat as part of this diet and plan your first week's menus.

Make a shopping list

Once you have decided what you are going to eat in the following week, make a shopping list of what you need and stick to it. Don't buy anything that is outside that list even if it is on special offer. Having fridge shelves full of special-offer yogurts will only tempt you to eat them before they pass their 'best-before' date.

With the exception of oily fish and oats, try to only buy foods with 5% or less fat as this will save you hundreds of calories. Look, too, for low-Gi options such as basmati rice in preference to other types, oat-based or high-fibre cereals, wholegrain bread with bits in it, pitta bread and pasta, and sweet or new potatoes in preference to old ones.

Plan your exercise schedule

We rarely 'feel like exercising' and so we are more likely to actually do it if we have made an exercise or activity schedule. This gives us a focus and means it's harder to make excuses to get out of it. If you want fast results and a great body, with taut skin, at the end of your diet and fitness campaign, you will need to do some aerobic exercise for 30 minutes on five days a week. Work out at a level of activity that makes you slightly breathless; e.g. aerobic dancing, brisk walking, strong swimming or light jogging. Do this and your inches and your weight will drop faster than you ever thought possible.

Try to add in some exercise sessions with a 'toning' or 'resistance' band to strengthen your muscles as you lose weight. This will help to improve your posture as well as tone your muscles and re-define your figure to give you a lovely shape.

Take some 'before' photographs

Ask a friend or partner to take 'before' photographs of you from the front, side, and back views and keep them somewhere safe. You don't have to show them to anyone else, but, when you are slim and look back at these photos, you'll be so glad that you took them.

Weigh and measure yourself

Weigh and measure yourself before you start the diet and keep a record on the charts at the back of this book. Take the widest measurement around your thighs, bust and hip bones. Also measure the widest part around your hips (if different) and just above the knees. Take the narrowest measurement around your upper arms and your waist. Men should measure around their abdomen, not underneath it where their trousers sit.

Get support

Whenever we take on a challenge we need support and encouragement. Who is going to support you? If you have a partner who will take delight in your progress and comfort you when the going gets tough, that's perfect. Getting together with other, like-minded dieters can be a huge help, too.

If there's a Rosemary Conley class in your area, do go along as all our instructors are professionally qualified to teach exercise and nutrition and there's the added bonus that you can be weighed on the same professional scales at the same time each week so that you get a very accurate check on your progress, plus you'll enjoy the support from fellow class members and do a fun workout all at the same class.

If there is no class near you, then why not try our online weight-loss club? See the back of this book for details.

Now you have acknowledged WHY you want to lose weight, hopefully you have decided to commit to doing it. So, read on.

5

Motivation – The Key to Success

We know if we are to lose weight, we have to eat fewer calories than our body spends in energy. And if we do extra exercise, we will burn more calories and lose weight faster. It's a matter of physics and relatively simple. The big problem is *motivation*. Finding the willpower to stick to the diet when the going gets tough can be a challenge!

Tempting times

When we start a diet we have bags of motivation and no-one can tempt us away from our resolve to eat less and do more. After about four weeks, though, we begin to find the odd crack in our up-to-now faultless determination and it doesn't take long before a few bad habits start to creep back in. The annoying thing is that it takes only a few lapses in willpower for the inevitable extra calories to sneak into our daily diet and cause our weight loss to come to a standstill.

We know we have cheated, yet we step on the scales and somehow expect a miracle to happen, hoping that we have still lost weight! Of course the miracle doesn't happen, so we become despondent and what follows is the inevitable relapse in our resolve. This is our most dangerous time. If we don't contain this, it can lead to a total collapse of our weight-loss campaign and we will gain weight and feel a huge sense of failure.

Positive thoughts

The key to success is keeping the motivation going, anticipating the hard times and being prepared for temptation to come knocking on our door. We must develop a really positive mental attitude in order to overcome any hitches and help us stay focused on the fantastically healthy, slim and fit body we are aiming for. And YES, it is there for the taking.

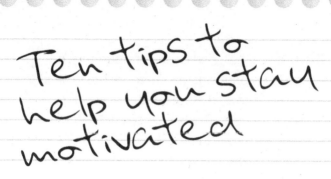

Ten tips to help you stay motivated

1 Weigh yourself once a week only and on the same scales, in the same clothes and at the same time of day. Write down your weight and use the graph at the back of this book to plot your progress.

2 Measure yourself weekly and keep a record, using the chart at the back of this book. Sometimes the inches reduce even when the scales don't budge!

3 Each week add your inch losses together and colour in the chart at the back of the book to help you realise just how many inches and how much weight you are losing.

4 Keep a carrier bag in a cupboard to fill each week with items of equal weight to that you have lost during the past seven days. Remind yourself of your ongoing achievement by lifting the bag often.

5 Use an old belt, skirt or pair of trousers as a physical progress guide. Keep a notepad nearby and write down the date and any relevant comments, e.g. 'Did belt up one notch today. Felt great. Really getting there now!' The more you remind yourself of your good feelings each time you try on your measuring garment as you lose weight, the more positive you will become. Make it a rule not to write down anything negative.

6 Write down activities for you to aim to do every day – even if it is only walking up and down stairs eight times while the adverts are on TV! Try walking to school/work/the pub/into town occasionally. Take up a sport. Work out to a fitness DVD. Play football/tennis/cricket with the children. Every little bit counts, leading to greater calorie-burning and faster results. You will be amazed at the direct correlation between activity and weight loss. The weeks you are more active will be the weeks you lose most weight.

7 Set yourself a physical challenge such as running the Race for Life, or perhaps be more ambitious and try a half marathon or even a full one. Training for an event adds a purpose to our exercise sessions, and makes them even more worthwhile.

8 Set yourself some short-term goals and then reward yourself when you reach each one, such as buying some special make-up or having your hair coloured. Try to delay buying too many new clothes until you reach your goal so that they have a longer life. Each time you reach a goal, ask your partner to put money into a separate account for your 'new wardrobe'!

9 Take photographs of yourself along your weight-loss journey. It will give you a real boost to compare yourself to them as you lose more weight.

10 Plan to do something really special to celebrate reaching your ultimate goal. Perhaps book a special holiday or weekend away. If the goal is exciting enough, it will motivate you to achieve your dreams.

6

The Amazing Shrinking Body

Most women fall into one of three basic body shapes, which I describe in simple terms as 'apple', 'pear', or 'heart'. Which shape you are depends largely on your genes and this determines your body fat distribution. So when weight is gained, an 'apple' will store proportionately more fat on her stomach, a 'pear' will store more fat on her hips and thighs, and a 'heart' on her chest.

If you are very overweight, say 18 stone, and an 'apple' shape, then you will undoubtedly be carrying a great deal of fat on your stomach. If you were to lose a significant amount of weight, the worry is that you could be left with folds of skin because the abdominal skin has been excessively stretched over a period of years.

The good news is that, providing you take the right approach to your weight-loss programme, you could significantly reduce that risk and end up with a better body than you ever thought possible.

Eating a healthy, low-fat diet with a calorie allowance appropriate to your gender, age and weight and combining this with moderate aerobic exercise such as brisk walking and some muscle-strengthening exercises should encourage the skin to shrink back significantly, although it's unrealistic to imagine that you could achieve an Elle MacPherson-style flat stomach (who of us could?). Just follow the advice below.

1 Eat enough

The worst thing would be to go on a crash diet of, say, 800 calories a day, as this would cause too rapid a weight loss and not help your skin to shrink back. Such a diet would, in effect, be 'starving' the body rather than 'feeding' it. Instead, following my Gi Hip and Thigh Diet with its brief Fat Attack Fortnight will get you off to a great start. Then you should move on to a more generous calorie allowance for the duration of your weight-loss programme. For a 40-year-old woman who weighed 18 stone, I would recommend a daily allowance of around 1700 calories, which is equal to her basal metabolic rate (BMR). That is the number of calories she would need each day for her body to function if she stayed in bed all day. As soon as she got up and went about her usual routine, every bit of activity she did would burn fat from her body. Result: weight, inch and fat loss at a healthy rate. As her weight decreases, she should reduce her daily allowance a little, so when she got down to, say, 11 stone, she should be eating around 1400 calories a day.

2 Check with your doctor

If you are carrying a great deal of excess weight, exercising is difficult for a number of reasons. Firstly, you will not be very mobile because your joints will struggle to cope with the heavy weight and your heart will have to work extremely hard when you start to move about. It is, therefore, important to get checked out by your doctor to see if you can start some gentle exercise without putting your health at risk.

3 Get moving

You need to do some aerobic exercise but don't be put off by the term 'aerobic'. Brisk walking is aerobic and what this type of exercise does is burn fat as fuel, which is exactly what you want. More than that, though, the increased oxygen that your body forces into your bloodstream when you start moving also reaches your skin, which will help it to shrink. All of this will help that tummy to reduce in size.

4 Start walking

The key is to start gently by walking just 200–300 metres. If you can do that a couple of times a day, that's brilliant. Gradually increase the distance and also look for opportunities to walk more in your everyday life. You will be amazed how those little journeys all mount up. When you are coping more easily, consider getting one of my fitness DVDs. Don't attempt the whole workout yet, but start with just the warm up. As you become fitter and more agile, progress to the next track. Before you finish, always fast-forward to the cool-down stretches and do these before you stop.

5 Do toning exercises

To increase the fat-burning effect, you will need to strengthen your muscles, particularly in this case, the abdominals. The fat burning that takes place during exercise only happens in the muscles and the bigger the muscles, the more effective the fat burning. Gradually increase the number of repetitions to further strengthen your muscles. If you are significantly over-weight, lying down on the floor can be uncomfortable, so it may be difficult to do abdominal exercises. Try placing a rolled-up towel under your head for support.

6 Apply cream

I am not for a moment suggesting that applying a cream to your skin is going to work miracles, because it won't, but there are two real benefits from using some kind of body lotion or baby oil every day after your bath or shower. When skin is significantly stretched, say during pregnancy or if you are seriously overweight, its elasticity is challenged. Applying a moisturising body lotion helps to keep skin soft and more pliable.

7 Massage your skin

In addition to replacing important moisture, the very act of applying body lotion massages the skin and helps improve cir-culation. This also encourages the skin to shrink back.

8 Improve your posture

Being very overweight can affect posture. Try to stand tall, draw your shoulders back, and lengthen your body. This will help to bring your body back in line if you have developed bad postural habits while carrying around your excess weight.

9 Pull in your stomach all the time!

I know it's a tall order but try to get into the habit of pulling in your tummy, any time, any place, anywhere! It is one of the best abdominal exercises and you can do it standing, sitting or lying. We already have the equivalent of a Playtex girdle built in to our bodies, but we need to *use* it to enjoy its full benefits. So stand tall, pull your tummy in and hold. Do this and your stomach will start taking on the shape it should be.

10 Drink plenty of water
This is a message we hear continually, but a very significant amount of our body weight is fluid and if you are dehydrated your body won't function properly. Drinking plenty of water helps skin stay healthy and flexible and is vital to helping your skin contract.

The result?

Follow these ten simple steps and you should lose around 2–3lb each week and your body will shrink naturally. Within months, your body will be transformed. As you become slimmer and fitter, keep up the aerobic and toning exercises and try to increase the amount of activity you do. The benefits to your health from exercising regularly are enormous, and investing just 20–30 minutes, five days a week, could save your life, let alone the cost of cosmetic surgery!

7

Eating for Good Health

In order for our bodies to function at their optimum level, we need to feed them a variety of essential nutrients. These fall into five basic categories – protein, carbohydrate, vitamins, minerals and fat.

We need protein for growth and repair, carbohydrates for energy, vitamins and minerals to boost our immune system and help cells and organs do their job. Lastly, we need some fat, also for energy.

Protein

Protein is vital for growth and repair of our body tissues. It is found in foods such as meat, fish, eggs, cheese and milk, and in non-animal sources, such as soya beans. Protein is very satiating and helps you feel fuller for longer, so try to have a portion at each meal.

When following a low-fat diet, always go for lean cuts of meat and trim away any visible fat. Remove the skin from poultry and choose low-fat cheeses and skimmed or semi-skimmed milk in preference to full fat. Choosing low-fat protein foods does not in any way reduce their nutritional content but it does reduce the number of calories dramatically and will also benefit your heart. The only exception is oily fish, as this contains essential fatty acids that are important for good health. So, aim to eat two portions a week of oily fish, such as mackerel, herring, or salmon.

Carbohydrates

Carbohydrates provide energy and can also give us a sense of fullness after eating them. As carbohydrates are very easily burned by the body, they are not readily stored as body fat. Carbohydrate foods include bread, potatoes, rice, pasta and cereals.

On my Gi Hip and Thigh Diet I recommend you consume some carbohydrate with every meal. Choose natural sources in preference to refined ones where possible and follow the Gi guidelines in chapter 3.

Vitamins and minerals

Vitamins occur naturally in food and form part of the family of micronutrients. These are nutrients that are essential for good health but only needed in very small (micro) amounts. Other micronutrients are minerals, such as iron and calcium, or trace elements, such as iodine or silicon, which are needed in minute (trace) amounts in the body.

There are many different kinds of vitamins, but they fall into two main categories according to their chemical structure.

Some, such as the B group of vitamins or vitamin C, are water-soluble. As the name suggests, these vitamins dissolve in water and are excreted from the body in urine. You should eat some of these nutrients every day. Others, such as vitamins A, D, E and K, are fat-soluble and are more easily stored by the body, so you can balance out your nutrient needs over a few days.

There is no single food that is essential, but choosing a varied and balanced diet will help you to obtain all the vitamins you need.

Vitamin A

This is a group of vitamins and it includes beta-carotene, which can be converted in the body to vitamin A. Vitamin A is essential for the immune system, for skin health and for good eyesight, especially in dim light. Carrots are rich in beta-carotene, which could explain the old wives' tale that carrots help you see in the dark! Vitamin A is found in meat, especially liver, and oily fish, eggs and dairy produce. Beta-carotene occurs in yellow, orange and dark green fruit and vegetables such as mangoes, peppers, carrots and spinach.

There are some concerns that too much vitamin A may not be good for health. Large quantities during pregnancy can increase the risk of fetal abnormalities, and high intakes over many years may increase the risk of bone fractures in later life. Vitamin A is an antioxidant and it has been suggested that it may help reduce the risk of cancer. However, a study among smokers actually showed an increased risk of cancer in those taking vitamin A supplements.

If you eat liver or liver products such as pâté once a week, you are likely to be eating the recommended amount of vitamin A and it may be advisable not to eat liver more often and to avoid supplements containing vitamin A. The Department of Health in the UK recommends that pregnant women avoid eating liver because of the specific risks to the unborn baby. There is no need to limit your intake of fruit and vegetables rich in beta-carotene.

B Vitamins

This is a whole family of vitamins with a range of different functions. B vitamins help to make red blood cells, which carry oxygen around the body and also metabolise food to produce energy. B vitamins are found in a wide variety of foods, including cereals, meat and dairy products.

The B vitamin folic acid is found in many vegetables and fruits and may be added to some other foods, such as breakfast cereals. Women who are planning a pregnancy or who are in the first 12 weeks of pregnancy should take a folic acid supplement (400 micrograms per day) to reduce the risk of having a baby with spina bifida.

Vitamin C

Over the years vitamin C has been credited with curing everything from the common cold to cancer, and it is found in a wide variety of fruit and vegetables. Levels of vitamin C decrease while food is being stored, and vitamin C is easily destroyed by cooking. To maximise your intake, choose very fresh or frozen fruit and vegetables and eat raw where possible, or cook only lightly, ideally steaming them or cooking in the microwave.

Vitamin C is needed by every cell in the body, including skin, blood vessels and even bones. It is a powerful antioxidant and helps the body to fight infections. It also helps the body to absorb iron efficiently from the gut into the bloodstream. However, there is little evidence that more than the recommended 40 milligrams of vitamin C a day has any extra health benefits. High doses of vitamin C are simply excreted in urine.

Vitamin D

In theory the body can make all the vitamin D it needs through the action of sunlight on the skin. Vitamin D is essential for healthy bones, and low intakes can lead to rickets in children or osteomalacia (a bone disease) in older people. Vitamin D is found in dairy foods, egg yolks, fatty fish and fish with small edible bones, such as sardines. Some foods, such as margarine, breakfast cereals and bread, are fortified with vitamin D. Liver is a good source of vitamin D, but it is best not to consume this more than once a week because it contains high levels of vitamin A.

Most people can get all the vitamin D they need from their diet or exposure to sun, but research shows that some groups of people may be at risk of vitamin D deficiency. The Department of Health in the UK recommends that pregnant or lactating women, and older people who are most at risk of deficiency, could usefully take a vitamin D supplement of 10 micrograms a day. If you spend little time outdoors, apply lots of sun cream or are of Asian origin, you may also benefit from a similar supplement.

Vitamin E

Vitamin E is best known as an antioxidant which helps protect the cells of the body from damage. It is found in vegetable oils, wholegrains, nuts and seeds.

Vitamin K

This is one of the lesser-known nutrients. It is essential for efficient blood clotting, and research suggests it is also vital for good bone health. Vitamin K is found in green vegetables and in some vegetable oils. It is also produced by some bacteria in the gut.

Do you need a vitamin supplement?

National surveys in the UK show that most people eat the recommended quantities of vitamins and do not require extra supplements. However, as an insurance policy, especially if you are dieting, you may wish to take a general multi-vitamin supplement. Choose a product with a wide range of vitamins, rather than single nutrients. Check the label to choose one that provides about the recommended intake of the different vitamins.

Consider taking a multi-vitamin supplement if you:

* are dieting
* have a poor appetite
* have erratic eating habits
* are a fussy or picky eater
* eat fewer than five portions of fruit and vegetables a day.

Many people take fish oil supplements and these frequently include some of the fat-soluble vitamins. If you take more than one supplement, remember to add up the total amount of vitamin present. If you are pregnant, or have any medical condition, consult your doctor before taking any supplements as they may interfere with your condition or with other medications.

It is important to consume sufficient vitamins, but more is not better, and in some cases may even be harmful. Research repeatedly shows that people who eat a varied diet with plenty of fruit and vegetables tend to live longer, healthier lives, but there is no evidence that the same is true for supplement users. Remember that pills are a supplement – not a substitute – for a healthy diet.

Fat

While fat is important as part of a balanced, healthy diet, these days we need only a small amount, yet high-fat food is all around us – in vending machines, petrol stations, restaurants and supermarkets – ready to tempt us. Not only are we eating more fat but, unfortunately, we are also burning fewer calories because our lives are not as physically demanding as they were in years gone by.

As far as weight loss is concerned, it doesn't matter whether fat is saturated or polyunsaturated; if you eat it, it will still be stored as fat on your body. If you are suffering from heart disease, it is especially important to cut down on saturated fat. Do this, and your heart condition should also improve – even more so if you lose weight and take regular exercise. So, my simple advice is to eat low fat as a matter of course by selecting foods (except oily fish) that have 5 % or less fat. This ensures you won't be missing out on essential nutrients from fat. It's virtually impossible to eat too little fat, as many common foods, such as bread, include some fat.

A healthy diet

The menus in this book are healthy and designed to provide all the nutrients you need. When choosing your own meals, though, try to vary your choices so that you obtain a balanced intake of nutrients.

I have been eating low-fat foods for 20 years and I have never felt better. My regular health checks, which include blood testing, confirm that everything is in very good order, so I am speaking from personal experience as well as under the guidance of nutritional experts.

8

Diet Instructions – Read These First!

To maximise your weight- and inch-loss progress, the diet is divided into two phases. Phase 1 is quite strict but is only for two weeks. Phase 2 is more lenient and versatile as from Week 3, depending on your gender, age and weight, you are likely to be able to add puddings, alcohol and treats.

Phase 1: The Fat Attack Fortnight

Research has shown that dieters who experience significant weight losses early on in their dieting campaign are much more likely to stick with their weight-reducing programme in the long term. With this in mind, I have created the Fat Attack Fortnight diet, which allows you a breakfast, lunch and dinner each day plus two Power Snacks in the form of fruit to eat whenever you choose, though I recommend you eat them mid-morning and mid-afternoon to stave off hunger pangs.

Also each day you should consume 450ml/¾ pint of skimmed or semi-skimmed milk, which you can have on your breakfast cereal and in your teas and coffees during the day as these drinks are unrestricted, as are water and low-calorie drinks.

Just for the first two weeks give alcohol a miss. Also refrain from eating anything outside the diet. The stricter you are, the more weight you will lose.

Lunch usually includes a small salad. If you wish, the salad can be saved and eaten as an extra snack or with your main meal in the evening. The salad will count as one of your five-a-day fruit and/or vegetable portions of which you should aim to eat your full quota every day within your meal selections and your Power Snacks.

In chapter 9 you will find a 14-day Fat Attack Fortnight diet, together with weekly shopping lists designed to meet the needs of just one person. So, if you are cooking and preparing meals for the whole family, you will need to modify the lists. There is also a daily activity challenge to help get you moving and burn extra calories.

If you prefer, for this Fat Attack Fortnight diet you can substitute any of the breakfast, lunch or dinner suggestions in Chapter 11.

Phase 2: The Gi Hip and Thigh Diet

By Week 3, if you have stuck strictly to the diet plan, you will be probably half a stone lighter and ready to eat more! At this stage, it is important to determine your BMR (basal metabolic rate), which you can do by checking the charts on pages 289–291. Simply look at the column against your gender, age and current weight. This is the number of calories your body uses each day just to stay alive.

Personal calorie allowance

To achieve your optimum rate of weight loss in Phase 2, I recommend you eat the equivalent number of calories to your BMR each day. This means that your body will be given sufficient food to fuel its basic needs, then every bit of activity you do, from stepping out of bed in the morning to going to work all day, will be fuelled by your fat stores. And the more activity you do, the more fat you will burn off your body and the quicker you will lose weight and look slimmer. So make every effort to do the daily activity challenge.

Extras

Once you have determined your personal BMR you will then see how many calories you have to 'spend' each day.

Throughout this book all the breakfasts are based on 200 calories, lunches are around 300 and dinners are 400 calories. This means that you can choose any of them to suit your individual preference.

So, for example, if you have a BMR/calorie allowance of around 1500 a day you can eat any breakfast, lunch and dinner from this book, include your 450ml/¾ pint milk allowance and two Power Snacks and then ADD a 100-calorie dessert, an alcoholic drink worth 100 calories and a 100-calorie treat which can be outside of the low-Gi, low-fat guidelines.

Make the diet work for you, so for instance, if you don't drink alcohol, you can use your calories elsewhere. If you want to drink two glasses of wine and not have a treat – you can. If you don't enjoy desserts, have an extra portion of rice, pasta or potatoes with your main meal instead. It is this versatility that will determine your long-term success.

If you have a lot of weight to lose and have, say, a BMR of 1800, then rather than using your 'extra' calories on alcohol and treats, it would be preferable to increase your portion sizes at meal times. My portion pots will help you to be accurate in estimating your portion sizes.

Diet Notes

Drinks
Regular and fruit teas and coffee made with water are unrestricted. Use milk from your daily allowance as required. Water is also unrestricted. Aim to drink 2 litres a day. All low-calorie drinks may be drunk freely.

Sugar
Calories from sugar and reduced-calorie sugar substitutes (such as Silver Spoon Half Spoon) should be counted into your daily calorie allowance.

Milk
Skimmed or semi-skimmed milk is recommended, but anyone allergic to or intolerant of cow's milk may have soya or rice milk. If you don't drink much milk you can swap 150ml milk for 125ml low-fat yogurt providing it has no more than 75 calories.

Bread
Low-Gi bread is made from stoneground or wholegrain flour. Check the nutrition panel on pre-packed loaves to find the calories per slice. In this diet 1 slice of bread has 100 calories.

Breakfast cereals

Choose oat-based or high-fibre varieties, e.g. All-Bran, Fruit 'n Fibre, Bran Buds, Grapenuts, muesli, or Shredded Wheat. Special K is also low Gi, and Weetabix is a good low-fat, low-sugar option.

Fruit

Aim to eat five portions of fruit or vegetables each day. A portion of fruit is one small orange, apple or pear or a regular nectarine or peach or 115g fruit such as berries or grapes. In the diet plans this is described as '1 piece fresh fruit'.

Vegetables

A 115g serving of vegetables counts as one of your five-a-day portions. All vegetables should be cooked and served without added fat. 'Unlimited vegetables' means any vegetables except potatoes.

Potatoes

Cook and eat new potatoes in their skins as this retains important fibre and reduces their Gi rating.

Salad

Salad includes all salad leaves, cress, tomatoes and raw vegetables such as cucumber, peppers, carrots, onion, mushrooms, celery and courgettes, and may be served with any low-calorie, oil-free dressing, balsamic vinegar or soy sauce. Avoid pre-packed or ready-made salads which include dressing as most are high in fat.

Oily fish

For good heart health it is important to eat two portions a week of oily fish, e.g. mackerel, salmon, sardines, herrings. Therefore, even though its fat content exceeds the 5% ruling, oily fish should still be included on a low-fat diet.

Fat grams and % fat

The rule of thumb I use in my diets is that all foods, bar a few exceptions, should contain no more than 5% fat. Food labels always state the nutrition values, so check them before you buy and only select foods with 5 grams or less per 100 grams of product. Even if you will be eating 300 grams of that product, say in the case of a ready meal, and consuming 15 grams of fat in total, then that is fine, as it is still a low-fat dish. This is a very easy and effective system of ensuring that, overall, you will be eating a low-fat diet.

Oats and dry powders

Porridge oats have more than 5% fat, but by the time you have cooked them with water and made them into porridge, the fat content will be minimal. The same applies to muesli. Adding skimmed or semi-skimmed milk or fruit juice brings the fat content well below the 5% mark. Also, foods such as custard powder, once reconstituted with milk or water, will be well within the 5% ruling.

Olive oil

Although olive oil is beneficial for the heart, it is still 100% fat, which is not good for your weight-loss campaign. You will already be doing a lot to help your heart quite naturally by losing weight, getting fitter and eating a low-fat diet, which will improve your cholesterol levels and blood pressure. You do not need to add oil to the food you eat to be healthy.

Olive oil sprays

These are helpful for people who still like to use just a little oil in their cooking, and cooking sprays deliver the tiniest amount of oil to your pan or food, which is useful for browning or crisping. As long as you count the calories into your daily total, the occasional spray will not do any harm.

Gravy

Make gravy with gravy powder or low-fat granules. I mix a little Bisto powder with some cold water, add the cooking water from vegetables, then bring to the boil for a few minutes – and the gravy tastes delicious. When roasting a joint of meat or a chicken, I always cook them on a rack in a roasting tin and then pour the remaining juices and sediment from the bottom of the tin into a fat separator jug. I can then pour the fat-free juices from the meat into the gravy to add flavour while the fat drains away.

Ⓥ means suitable for vegetarians or vegetarian option is available.

❋ means suitable for freezing.

9

The Fat Attack Fortnight

Follow this diet plan for two weeks – and lose weight fast! Then move on to Phase 2. Remember, you can substitute any breakfast, lunch or dinner from chapter 11. Always do the daily activity challenge to ensure you achieve your optimum weight loss.

All the diet menus are designed for just one person and a shopping list has been created for each week's eating plan. Check through the plans to see if all the meal suggestions are ones you will enjoy. If not, substitute alternatives from chapter 11 and adjust your shopping list accordingly. If you are preparing meals for more than one person you will also need to amend the list.

I have included the appropriate Rosemary Conley Portion Pot colour in the menu plans to help you measure portion sizes with greater ease and accuracy, but in case you do not yet own a set, I have also given the equivalent metric weight equivalents.

Week 1 Diet

DAILY ALLOWANCE

450ml/¾ pint skimmed or semi-skimmed milk	200 kcal
Breakfast	200 kcal
Mid-morning Power Snack	50 kcal
Lunch	300 kcal
Mid-afternoon Power Snack	50 kcal
Dinner	400 kcal
Total	1200 kcal

Day One

Breakfast

1 yellow portion pot/125ml fresh orange juice plus 1 red portion pot/40g Special K cereal served with milk from allowance and 1 tsp sugar Ⓥ

Mid-morning Power Snack

1 small pear

Lunch

1 medium wholemeal pitta bread filled with 1 tbsp tomato salsa, a handful of rocket leaves, sliced cucumber and 50g sliced cooked chicken (no skin)

Mid-afternoon Power Snack

1 nectarine or peach

Dinner

1 × 150g tuna steak, sprinkled with black pepper and lime juice, grilled, and served with 1 blue portion pot/55g (uncooked weight) or 1 red portion pot/144g (cooked weight) basmati rice, plus chopped vegetables (½ each red, green and yellow peppers, beansprouts, ½ red onion, 1 carrot) dry-fried with a little soy sauce

ACTIVITY CHALLENGE

- Walk briskly for 20 minutes

- Do 2 × 8 reps of ab curls: Lie on back with knees bent and feet hip width apart. Place hands behind head to support neck. Lift head and shoulders off floor, pulling tummy in tight. Lower again slowly, keeping tummy in

Day Two

Breakfast
1 slice toasted wholegrain bread topped with 1 yellow portion pot/115g baked beans; 1 piece fresh fruit Ⓥ

Mid-morning Power Snack
75g seedless grapes

Lunch
300ml fresh or 1 × 400g can tomato soup (max. 150 kcal and 5% fat) served with 1 slice toasted wholegrain bread and a small salad Ⓥ

Mid-afternoon Power Snack
1 apple

Dinner
Pork and Pineapple Kebabs (see recipe, page 191) served with a little sweet chilli dipping sauce and 200g steamed green vegetables or a mixed salad

ACTIVITY CHALLENGE

• Walk briskly for 10 minutes

• Walk up and down stairs 3 times consecutively

• Do 10 minutes of toning exercises from this book (see pages 255–63) or from a fitness DVD

Day Three

Breakfast

½ melon filled with 1 red portion pot/115g raspberries and topped with 1 low-fat yogurt (max. 100 kcal and 5% fat) Ⓥ

Mid-morning Power Snack

1 peach or nectarine

Lunch

1 slice toasted wholegrain bread topped with 150g drained, canned tuna in brine mixed with 1 tsp extra light mayonnaise, 1 blue portion pot/80g 0% fat Greek-style yogurt (e.g. Total 0%) and lemon juice, served with a small salad

Mid-afternoon Power Snack

2 satsumas

Dinner

1 × 175g chicken breast (no skin) wrapped in foil and cooked under the grill for 15 minutes, turning occasionally to ensure that the chicken is thoroughly cooked. Serve with 115g boiled sweet potatoes and unlimited green vegetables of your choice plus gravy made from gravy powder or low-fat granules

ACTIVITY CHALLENGE

• Do 30 minutes of aerobic exercise (work out at a class, to an aerobics or salsacise fitness DVD or on cardio equipment at the gym)

Day Four

Breakfast
1 × 100g low-fat yogurt (max. 75 kcal and 5% fat) mixed with 1 tbsp unsweetened muesli and 1 red portion pot/115g raspberries Ⓥ

Mid-morning Power Snack
¼ melon

Lunch
1 egg, dry-fried, and 2 turkey rashers, grilled, served with unlimited grilled tomatoes and mushrooms and a small mixed salad

Mid-afternoon Power Snack
1 small pear

Dinner
1 yellow portion pot/45g (uncooked weight) or 1 red portion pot/110g (cooked weight) pasta shapes boiled with a vegetable stock cube and drained. Add ½ jar (approx. 200g) ready-made low-fat tomato and basil pasta sauce and heat through. Serve with chopped fresh basil leaves and a sprinkling of Parmesan shavings plus a large green salad Ⓥ

ACTIVITY CHALLENGE

- Walk briskly for 20 minutes

- Walk up and down stairs 3 times consecutively

- Do 2 × 10 reps of outer thigh toner (see page 257)

Day Five

Breakfast
Gi fruit salad: 1 satsuma, broken into segments, 1 chopped pear, 25g seedless grapes and 15g porridge oats. Mix with 1 blue portion pot/80g 0% fat Greek yogurt Ⓥ

Mid-morning Power Snack
¼ melon

Lunch
2 slices wholegrain bread spread with low-calorie salad dressing and made into a sandwich with 25g wafer thin ham, chicken, beef or turkey, plus a small salad

Mid-afternoon Power Snack
75g seedless grapes

Dinner
1 × 150g salmon steak, grilled, served with 115g boiled new potatoes (with skins) and a large mixed salad tossed in oil-free dressing plus 2 tsps sweet chilli dipping sauce

ACTIVITY CHALLENGE

• Do 25 minutes of brisk walking

• Do 6 tricep dips on stairs: Start with both hands resting on edge of stairs, and hips close to edge. Pull tummy in tight and bend elbows, lowering hips towards floor. Push up again, with shoulders down, head up and avoid locking elbows

Day Six

Breakfast

1 blue portion pot/40g unsweetened muesli served with milk from allowance and 1 chopped nectarine or peach Ⓥ

Mid-morning Power Snack

1 apple

Lunch

1 × 175g baked sweet potato topped with 1 yellow portion pot/115g baked beans and served with grilled mushrooms, plus a small salad Ⓥ

Mid-afternoon Power Snack

2 satsumas

Dinner

1 × 150g chicken breast (no skin), grilled, served with 1 blue portion pot/55g (uncooked weight) or 1 red portion pot/144g (cooked weight) basmati rice plus tomato and pepper sauce (dry-fry ½ red onion, chopped, with ½ each red, green and yellow peppers, add 1 small can chopped tomatoes, a dash of Worcestershire sauce and season with black pepper. Boil until reduced slightly and add fresh basil if desired)

ACTIVITY CHALLENGE

• Do 30 consecutive minutes of energetic housework, gardening or car washing

• Do 10 minutes of toning exercises from this book (see pages 255–63) or from a fitness DVD

Day Seven

Breakfast

1 blue portion pot/40g unsweetened muesli soaked overnight with 1 blue portion pot/80ml unsweetened apple juice. Serve with 1 tsp 0% fat Greek yogurt Ⓥ

Mid-morning Power Snack

1 small pear

Lunch

Leek, Pea, Smoked Ham and Cheese Pasta (see recipe, page 195) served with a small salad

Mid-afternoon Power Snack

75g seedless grapes

Dinner

115g thinly sliced roast chicken or turkey (all fat and skin removed) or 150g Quorn Chicken Style Roast served with 115g dry-roast sweet potatoes, 75g dry-roast parsnips and unlimited other vegetables plus low-fat gravy Ⓥ

ACTIVITY CHALLENGE

• Do 30 minutes of aerobic exercise (work out at a class, to a fitness DVD, or on cardio equipment at the gym), or play an outdoor game such as football or tennis for 30–40 minutes

• Do 2 × 6 reps of press-ups:
Position yourself on hands and knees, hands in line with shoulders and knees directly under hips. Pull tummy in to support back and then bend elbows, taking forehead towards floor. Lift up again without locking elbows at top

Week 1 Shopping List

Store cupboard items
extra light mayonnaise
low-fat gravy granules/gravy powder
low-fat salad dressing (e.g. Waistline) plus oil-free dressing
low-fat tomato salsa or relish
maple syrup
pasta shapes
rice (basmati)
salt and freshly ground black pepper
soy sauce
sugar (or Silver Spoon Half Spoon)
sweet chilli dipping sauce
vegetable stock cubes
Worcestershire sauce

Breakfast cereals and bread
porridge oats
Special K
unsweetened muesli
1 sliced wholegrain loaf
1 pack wholemeal pitta bread (1 pitta needed – freeze
    remainder for subsequent weeks)

Canned and frozen foods
1 × 200g can tuna in brine
1 × 230g can baked beans
1 × 200g can chopped tomatoes
1 × 400g can or 300ml fresh tomato soup (max. 5% fat)
1 small can or jar/200g tomato and basil pasta sauce

1 small bag frozen peas

Dairy
2.8 litres/5 pints skimmed or semi-skimmed milk
6 eggs (1 needed – use remainder in subsequent weeks)
1 small pot yogurt (max. 100 kcal and 5 % fat)
1 small pot yogurt (max. 75 kcal and 5 % fat)
2 × 150g pots 0 % fat Greek-style yogurt
1 × 200g pot Philadelphia Extra Light soft cheese (50g
     needed – use remainder in subsequent weeks)
Parmesan cheese (100g will last several weeks)

Fresh meat and fish
1 × 175g chicken breast plus 1 × 150g chicken breast
1 × 150g fresh salmon steak
1 × 150g tuna steak
1 × 150g lean pork steak
1 slice smoked ham
50g cooked chicken breast plus 115g thinly sliced roast
     chicken or turkey (or 150g Quorn Chicken Style Roast)
25g wafer thin meat (ham, chicken, turkey or beef)
1 pack turkey rashers (2 rashers needed – freeze rest)

Fresh fruit
1 melon
230g raspberries
2 apples
3 nectarines or peaches
4 small pears
5 satsumas
250g seedless grapes

1 lemon plus 1 lime
1 small pack fresh pineapple chunks
1 piece fresh fruit of your choice

Fresh fruit juice
apple juice (80ml)
orange juice (125ml)

Fresh vegetables and salad items
1 carrot
1 green, 1 red and 1 yellow pepper
1 red onion
3 large tomatoes plus 1 pack cherry tomatoes
1 pack mushrooms
2 baby leeks
75g parsnips
200g green vegetables of your choice
extra mixed vegetables (enough for 2 portions)
115g new potatoes
230g sweet potatoes (for boiling)
1 × 175g sweet potato (for baking)
1 pack beansprouts
1 pack celery
1 cucumber
1 pack mixed salad leaves plus 1 pack rocket leaves
1 bunch spring onions

Fresh herbs and spices
basil leaves
1 garlic bulb
1 small red chilli

Week 2 Diet

Well done if you successfully completed Week 1 of the diet and managed to do all the daily activity challenges. You will be looking and feeling slimmer and will have already increased your level of fitness. Now for Week 2!

If you haven't yet sent off for a set of Rosemary Conley Portion Pots, I strongly recommend that you do. Accurate portion control is the key to your success and the portion pots will make that so much easier.

The daily activity challenges will enable you to build on the increased fitness you have already achieved. It is crucial that you do them each day if you want to achieve maximum weight loss in the shortest possible time, in a healthy way. The exercises will also you tone you up as you slim down.

Remember to check thorough next week's menus and amend your shopping list if you want to substitute any meals from chapter 11 or if you are preparing meals for more than one person.

DAILY ALLOWANCE

450ml/¾ pint skimmed or semi-skimmed milk	200 kcal
Breakfast	200 kcal
Mid-morning Power Snack	50 kcal
Lunch	300 kcal
Mid-afternoon Power Snack	50 kcal
Dinner	400 kcal
Total	1200 kcal

Day Eight

Breakfast
1 egg, poached or dry-fried, served with 2 grilled turkey rashers and unlimited grilled tomatoes

Mid-morning Power Snack
1 apple

Lunch
1 × 400g can any lentil or vegetable soup (max. 200 kcal and 5% fat) topped with a swirl of low-fat yogurt and served with 1 slice wholegrain bread or small wholegrain roll, plus a small salad (V)

Mid-afternoon Power Snack
100g mangoes or cherries

Dinner
1 × 175g salmon steak, grilled, served with 115g boiled new potatoes (with skins) and unlimited green vegetables (V)

ACTIVITY CHALLENGE

• Take 2 × 15-minute brisk walks during the day

• Do 15 minutes of toning exercises from this book (see pages 255–63) or from a fitness DVD

Day Nine

Breakfast
1 small banana, sliced, mixed with 115g sliced strawberries and 1 × 100g pot low-fat yogurt (max. 100 kcal and 5 % fat) Ⓥ

Mid-morning Power Snack
1 orange

Lunch
50g cooked chicken breast (no skin), chopped, mixed with 1 tbsp each low-fat yogurt and mango chutney and served on 2 Dark Rye Ryvita crispbreads, plus a small salad

Mid-afternoon Power Snack
2 kiwi fruits

Dinner
Chicken with Lime and Ginger (see recipe, page 152) served with 1 blue portion pot/55g (uncooked weight) or 1 red portion pot/144g (cooked weight) basmati rice

ACTIVITY CHALLENGE

• Walk up and down stairs 4 times twice during the day

• Do 3 × 6 reps of tricep dips on the stairs (see Day 5, page 56)

Day Ten

Breakfast
1 × 35g Rosemary Conley Low Gi Nutrition Bar and
2 pieces fresh fruit Ⓥ

Mid-morning Power Snack
1 apple

Lunch
Rice salad: Mix 1 blue portion pot/55g (uncooked
weight) or 1 red portion pot/144g (cooked weight)
basmati rice with chopped spring onions, diced
peppers, 1 tbsp canned sweetcorn, 1 segmented,
peeled orange and 2 tbsps oil-free salad dressing.
Serve with a small mixed salad Ⓥ

Mid-afternoon Power Snack
100g mangoes or cherries

Dinner
Any ready meal (max. 400 kcal
and 5% fat) Ⓥ

ACTIVITY CHALLENGE

• Do 40 minutes of aerobic
exercise (work out at a class,
to a fitness DVD or on cardio
equipment at the gym)

• Do 2 × 10 reps of bottom
tightener (see page 258)

Day Eleven

Breakfast

1 × 200g pot Rosemary Conley Ready to Eat Porridge
plus 1 kiwi fruit OR 1 blue portion pot/35g porridge oats
cooked with water and served with milk from allowance,
1 tsp honey or sugar and 1 piece fresh fruit Ⓥ

Mid-morning Power Snack

1 small banana

Lunch

Chicken Caesar salad: 1 Little Gem lettuce tossed with
chopped cucumber chunks, 115g sliced cooked
chicken breast (no skin) mixed with 4 tsps low-fat
Caesar dressing (max. 5% fat) and topped with a few
Parmesan shavings and home-made garlic croutons
(1 × 2cm slice wholegrain baguette rubbed with cut
clove of garlic, then cut into quarters and slowly
toasted under preheated grill until golden brown)

Mid-afternoon Power Snack

2 kiwi fruits

Dinner

1 small low-fat pizza (max. 350
kcal and 5% fat) served with a
mixed salad Ⓥ

ACTIVITY CHALLENGE

• Walk briskly for 30 minutes

• Walk up and down stairs 4
times consecutively

• Do 3 × 8 reps of ab curls
(see Day 1, page 52)

Day Twelve

Breakfast

1 Weetabix or Shredded Wheat served with milk from allowance, 1 tsp sugar and 1 thinly sliced small banana Ⓥ

Mid-morning Power Snack

1 orange

Lunch

2 low-fat beef or pork sausages (max. 5% fat) or 2 Quorn sausages, grilled, served on 1 slice toasted wholegrain bread with 1 × 200g can tomatoes boiled until thick and reduced, plus a small salad Ⓥ

Mid-afternoon Power Snack

1 small banana

Dinner

200g steamed white fish served with 115g boiled new potatoes plus unlimited vegetables of your choice and 100ml low-fat parsley sauce (made with skimmed milk)

ACTIVITY CHALLENGE

• Do 30 minutes of aerobics by working out at a class, to a fitness DVD or at the gym

• Do 8 press-ups twice during the day (see Day 7, page 58)

Day Thirteen

Breakfast

½ pink grapefruit, plus 1 slice toasted wholegrain bread spread with 2 tsps honey, jam or marmalade Ⓥ

Mid-morning Power Snack

1 apple

Lunch

1 small wholegrain roll spread with horseradish sauce, filled with 50g wafer thin beef and sliced tomatoes, plus a small salad

Mid-afternoon Power Snack

100g mangoes or cherries

Dinner

2 low-fat beef or pork sausages (max. 5% fat) or 2 Quorn sausages, grilled, served with 1 yellow portion pot/100g mashed sweet potatoes plus unlimited vegetables of your choice and low-fat gravy; 1 Rosemary Conley Low Fat Belgian Chocolate Mousse or 2 pieces fresh fruit Ⓥ

ACTIVITY CHALLENGE

• Do 30 minutes of energetic chores such as car washing, housework or gardening

• Play an energetic game, such as football, with the children for 15 minutes or go for a 20-minute brisk walk or bike ride

Day Fourteen

Breakfast

½ whole pink grapefruit; 1 medium-sized poached egg served on 1 slice toasted wholegrain bread Ⓥ

Mid-morning Power Snack

1 orange

Lunch

1 small wholegrain roll spread with 25g Philadelphia Extra Light soft cheese and filled with 25g smoked salmon, plus a small salad

Mid-afternoon Power Snack

1 apple

Dinner

75g roast beef served with either 1 low-fat Yorkshire pudding or 75g dry-roasted sweet potatoes, plus unlimited green vegetables and low-fat gravy

ACTIVITY CHALLENGE

• Walk briskly for 40 minutes or more leisurely for an hour

• Do 10 minutes of toning exercises from this book (see pages 255–63) or from a fitness DVD

Week 2 Shopping List

Store cupboard items
(in addition to Week 1)
chicken stock cubes

cornflour (if making fresh parsley sauce)

ground cumin

ground ginger

horseradish sauce

jam, honey or marmalade

lemongrass paste

low-fat Caesar salad dressing (max. 5% fat)

mango chutney

parsley sauce mix (or make fresh)

Breakfast cereals and bread
Weetabix or Shredded Wheat

1 box Rosemary Conley Low Gi Nutrition Bars (available from
www.rosemaryconley.com or Rosemary Conley Clubs)

1 pack Dark Rye Ryvita crispbreads

1 sliced wholegrain loaf

2 small wholegrain rolls

1 small wholegrain baguette (for croutons)

Canned foods
1 × 400g can lentil or vegetable soup (max. 200 kcal and
5% fat)

1 × 200g can chopped tomatoes

1 small can sweetcorn

Dairy
2.8 litres/5 pints skimmed or semi-skimmed milk
2 eggs (use ones bought in Week 1)
1 small pot low-fat natural yogurt (max. 5% fat)
1 small pot low-fat yogurt (max. 100 kcal and 5% fat),
    any flavour
75g Philadelphia Extra Light soft cheese (use leftover cheese
    from Week 1)

Fresh meat and fish
1 × 150g chicken breast
1 × 175g salmon steak
200g white fish (e.g. cod)
2 turkey rashers (or use from pack bought in Week 1)
4 low-fat beef or pork sausages (max. 5% fat) or 4 Quorn
    sausages
50g wafer thin beef
75g thinly sliced roast beef
165g cooked chicken breast
25g smoked salmon

From the chiller cabinet
1 pot Rosemary Conley Ready To Eat Porridge (available from
    Morrisons or Asda), or make your own porridge, using oats
    bought in Week 1
1 pack Rosemary Conley Low Fat Belgian Chocolate Mousse
    (or 2 extra pieces fresh fruit)
1 low-fat ready meal (max. 400 kcal and 5% fat)
1 low-fat pizza (max. 350 kcal and 5% fat)
1 low-fat Yorkshire pudding (or 75g sweet potatoes – see
    Day 14)

Fresh fruit

4 apples
4 small bananas
1 pink grapefruit
5 kiwi fruits
1 lime
4 oranges
300g mangoes or cherries
115g strawberries
3 pieces fresh fruit of your choice

Fresh vegetables and salad items

1 pack mixed salad leaves
1 Little Gem lettuce
1 pack cherry tomatoes
1 cucumber
3 large tomatoes
1 red, 1 green and 1 yellow pepper
1 white onion
1 baby leek
1 bunch spring onions
extra vegetables of your choice (enough for 4 portions)
230g new potatoes
175g sweet potatoes (or 1 low-fat Yorkshire pudding – see
    Day 14)

Fresh herbs and spices

coriander
parsley (if making fresh parsley sauce)
1 garlic bulb

The Gi Hip and Thigh Diet: Phase 2

10

If you have stuck rigidly to the Fat Attack Fortnight diet (Phase 1), you should be feeling significantly slimmer and fitter. Now, if your calorie allowance permits, it's time for some treats!

Before you start Phase 2, check your BMR in the charts on pages 288–91 to find your personal daily calorie allowance. Then, in addition to your three main meals a day and two Power Snacks, you may be able to have a dessert, a treat and an alcoholic drink each day, depending on your allowance.

On pages 75–81 you will find a two-week menu plan with shopping lists designed for one person. Use this if you wish to follow a set eating plan or, if you prefer, you can choose your own meals from the Gi Hip and Thigh Diet breakfast, lunch and dinner menu plans in chapter 11. Whether you follow the set menu plan or make your own choices, remember to add on your Power Snacks plus your dessert, treat and alcohol choices (see pages 132–139) according to your allowance. I have not included these in the menu plans or shopping lists for Week 3 and 4 because I don't know which ones you prefer and how you may wish to use your treat allowance. You can save up your treats over seven days for a special occasion if you want.

Make sure you use your daily 450ml/¾ pint milk allowance. You can drink as much water as you like – aim for at least 2 litres each day. Low-calorie soft drinks are also unlimited.

Week 3 Diet

DAILY ALLOWANCE

450ml/¾ pint skimmed or semi-skimmed milk	200 kcal
Breakfast	200 kcal
Mid-morning Power Snack	50 kcal
Lunch	300 kcal
Mid-afternoon Power Snack	50 kcal
Dinner	400 kcal
Total	1200 kcal

Plus optional extras (if calorie allowance permits):

Dessert	approx. 100 kcal
Treat	100 kcal
Alcohol	100 kcal

Day Fifteen

Breakfast
1 Müllerlight Corner Healthy Balance yogurt plus 5 sliced strawberries Ⓥ

Mid-morning Power Snack
½ × 35g Rosemary Conley Low Gi Nutrition Bar (eat remaining half on Day 17)

Lunch
1 small granary baguette filled with 50g diced, cooked beetroot, 50g smoked trout fillets plus watercress or rocket leaves, served with 1 blue portion pot/85g virtually fat-free fromage frais mixed with 1 tsp horseradish sauce

Mid-afternoon Power Snack
1 small banana

Dinner
Boozy Beef with Mushrooms (see recipe, page 171) served with 100g boiled new potatoes (with skins) plus a selection of other fresh vegetables

ACTIVITY CHALLENGE

• Work out to a fitness DVD for 40 minutes or attend a fitness class

Day Sixteen

Breakfast
1 yellow portion pot/50g unsweetened muesli with milk from allowance Ⓥ

Mid-morning Power Snack
1 Ryvita Dark Rye Crispbread with 50g low-fat salsa

Lunch
Chilli Bean Soup (see recipe, page 144) served with 1 slice wholegrain bread; 2 satsumas Ⓥ

Mid-afternoon Power Snack
150g strawberries with 1 tsp 0% fat Greek-style yogurt

Dinner
Spiced Tomato Baked Cod (see recipe, page 198) served with 1 blue portion pot/55g (uncooked weight) or 1 red portion pot/144g (cooked weight) basmati rice and seasonal vegetables or salad tossed in oil-free dressing

ACTIVITY CHALLENGE

• Walk up and down stairs 5 times consecutively

• Do 4 × 8 reps of ab curls (see Day 1, page 52)

• Do 3 × 6 reps of tricep dips (see Day 5, page 56)

Day Seventeen

Breakfast
Fruit salad made with 200g fresh seasonal berries and
1 blue portion pot/80ml unsweetened orange juice
topped with 1 tsp 0% fat Greek-style yogurt Ⓥ

Mid-morning Power Snack
½ × 35g Rosemary Conley Low Gi Nutrition Bar

Lunch
2 slices wholegrain bread, toasted, topped with
1 × 150g can baked beans Ⓥ

Mid-afternoon Power Snack
1 small banana

Dinner
115g braised lamb's liver
cooked with sliced onions and
gravy and served with 115g
boiled new potatoes (with
skins) and unlimited vegetables
of your choice

ACTIVITY CHALLENGE

• Take 2 brisk 20-minute
walks during the day

• Do 3 × 6 reps of press-ups
(see Day 7, page 58)

Day Eighteen

Breakfast
1 red portion pot/50g bran flakes served with milk from allowance and 1 tsp sugar Ⓥ

Mid-morning Power Snack
2 satsumas

Lunch
25g wafer thin ham, turkey or chicken served with a mixed salad tossed in oil-free dressing: 1 Rosemary Conley Low Gi Nutrition Bar and 1 small banana

Mid-afternoon Power Snack
2 kiwi fruits

Dinner
Sticky Onion Chicken (see recipe, page 151) served with 1 blue portion pot/55g (uncooked weight) or 1 red portion pot/144g (cooked weight) boiled basmati rice and salad

ACTIVITY CHALLENGE

• Work out to a fitness DVD for at least 40 minutes or attend a fitness class

Day Nineteen

Breakfast
1 red portion pot/50g Fruit 'n Fibre cereal served
with milk from allowance and 1 tsp sugar, plus
1 kiwi fruit Ⓥ

Mid-morning Power Snack
1 Dark Rye Ryvita Crispbread with 50g low-fat salsa

Lunch
1 low-fat beef or pork sausage (max. 5% fat) or
1 Quorn sausage, grilled, served with 1 yellow portion
pot/115g baked beans, 115g grilled mushrooms and
1 slice toasted wholegrain bread Ⓥ

Mid-afternoon Power Snack
2 satsumas

Dinner
1 × 175g tuna steak, grilled,
served with any low-fat relish or
tomato salsa plus 115g boiled
new potatoes (with skins) and
unlimited green vegetables

ACTIVITY CHALLENGE

• Take a 20-minute very brisk
walk or a bike ride

• Do 4 × 8 reps of ab curls
(see Day 1, page 52)

• Do 4 × 6 reps of press-ups
(see Day 7, page 58)

Day Twenty

Breakfast
1 yellow portion pot/125ml unsweetened fruit juice; 1 slice toasted wholegrain bread topped with 1 yellow portion pot/115g baked beans Ⓥ

Mid-morning Power Snack
1 small banana

Lunch
1 yellow portion pot/45g (uncooked weight) or 1 red portion pot/110g (cooked weight) boiled pasta shapes tossed with 50g smoked salmon strips and 1 yellow portion pot/135g virtually fat free fromage frais with chopped fresh dill, plus a green salad

Mid-afternoon Power Snack
1 Dark Rye Ryvita Crispbread with 50g low-fat salsa

Dinner
½ × 410g can Stagg Vegetable Garden Vegetable Chilli served with 1 blue portion pot/55g (uncooked weight) or 1 red portion pot/144g (cooked weight) boiled basmati rice, plus a small salad Ⓥ

Day Twenty-one

Breakfast

1 poached or dry-fried egg served with 1 low-fat beef or pork sausage (max. 5% fat) or 1 Quorn sausage, grilled, 3 grilled tomatoes and 100g grilled mushrooms Ⓥ

Mid-morning Power Snack

2 kiwi fruits

Lunch

½ × 410g can Stagg Vegetable Garden Vegetable Chilli and 1 small wholegrain roll plus a small salad Ⓥ

Mid-afternoon Power Snack

1 Dark Rye Ryvita Crispbread with 50g low-fat salsa

Dinner

Tomato and mushroom pasta: Dry-fry 175g sliced mushrooms lightly with ½ chopped onion and 1 crushed garlic clove. Stir in 1 × 200g can chopped tomatoes plus black pepper and chopped fresh basil. Meanwhile, cook 100g (uncooked weight) tagliatelle and combine with the tomato and mushroom mixture. Serve with steamed vegetables or salad Ⓥ

Week 3 Shopping List

All recipes serve one except for Boozy Beef with Mushrooms and Chilli Bean Soup, both of which serve 4 and can be frozen. Otherwise, if preparing meals for more than one person or substituting meals from chapter 11, you will need to amend the shopping list accordingly.

Store cupboard items (in addition to Weeks 1 and 2)
beef stock cubes
paprika
plain flour
runny honey
saffron
tagliatelle
tomato purée
turmeric

Breakfast cereals and bread
bran flakes
Fruit 'n Fibre
1 Rosemary Conley Low Gi Nutrition Bar from box bought in
   Week 2
1 small granary baguette
1 sliced wholegrain loaf
1 small wholegrain roll

Canned foods
1 × 150g can baked beans
1 × 250g can baked beans (230g required)
1 × 400g can chopped tomatoes

1 × 200g can plum tomatoes
1 × 200g can chickpeas
1 × 200g can red kidney beans
1 × 410g can Stagg Vegetable Garden Vegetable Chilli
300ml/½ pint stout, cider or beer

Dairy

2.8 litres/5 pints skimmed or semi-skimmed milk
1 egg (use one from Week 1)
1 small pot 0% fat Greek-style yogurt
1 × 220g pot virtually fat free fromage frais

Fresh meat and fish

25g wafer thin ham, chicken or turkey
1 × 175g chicken breast
115g lamb's liver
450g braising steak
2 low-fat beef or pork sausages (max. 5% fat)
    or 2 Quorn sausages
50g smoked salmon
50g smoked trout fillets
1 × 200g cod steak
1 × 175g tuna steak

From the chiller cabinet

1 Müllerlight Corner Healthy Balance yogurt (max. 5% fat)
200g low-fat tomato salsa (or use canned)

Fresh fruit

5 kiwi fruits
1 lemon plus 1 lime

4 small bananas
6 satsumas
200g strawberries
225g fresh mixed berries

Fresh fruit juice
fruit juice of your choice (125ml)
orange juice (80ml)

Fresh vegetables and salad items
4 large tomatoes
4 red onions plus 1 white onion
500g sliced mushrooms
50g cooked beetroot
extra vegetables of your choice (enough for 4 portions)
345g new potatoes
1 pack mixed salad leaves
1 pack watercress or rocket leaves
1 pack cherry tomatoes
1 cucumber
1 bunch spring onions
1 red or green pepper

Fresh herbs and spices
basil
dill
oregano
1 garlic bulb
1 small red chilli
fresh stem ginger

Week 4 Diet

If you have stuck strictly to this Gi Hip and Thigh Diet for the last three weeks and completed all the daily activity challenges, your clothes should be feeling very loose! Women may have dropped a whole dress size and men may have tightened their waist belts a couple of notches. How good does that make you feel? Now that you have achieved this much success in just three weeks, give it your very best effort in Week 4!

Use your portion pots for measuring basic foods. Stick to the meal suggestions and quantities given, whether you are following the set plan or choosing your own meals from the options in chapter 11. Use your dessert, treat and alcohol allowances wisely and accurately, and make sure you complete the daily activity challenges.

DAILY ALLOWANCE

450ml/¾ pint skimmed or semi-skimmed milk	200 kcal
Breakfast	200 kcal
Mid-morning Power Snack	50 kcal
Lunch	300 kcal
Mid-afternoon Power Snack	50 kcal
Dinner	400 kcal
Total	1200 kcal

Plus optional extras (if calorie allowance permits):
Dessert
Treat
Alcohol

Day Twenty-two

Breakfast
Fruity porridge: 1 blue portion pot/40g dry porridge oats, cooked in water, served with milk from allowance, ½ tsp honey or sugar or 1 pot Rosemary Conley Ready To Eat Porridge, plus 25g fresh seasonal berries Ⓥ

Mid-morning Power Snack
1 apple or pear

Lunch
1 × 150g chicken breast (no skin), grilled, served with a mixed salad

Mid-afternoon Power Snack
1 small banana

Dinner
1 × 175g oven-baked sweet potato topped with 100g canned tuna in brine, drained and mixed with 4 tsps low-fat salad dressing (e.g. Waistline), 25g canned sweetcorn and 2 tsps 0% fat Greek-style yogurt. Serve with a large salad

ACTIVITY CHALLENGE

• Do an aerobic workout for at least 40 minutes (work out at an aerobics class, to a fitness DVD or on cardio equipment at the gym). Increase the intensity now

Day Twenty-three

Breakfast

Turkey rasher sandwich: Spread 1 slice wholegrain bread with tomato ketchup, cut in half and make into a sandwich with 3 slices grilled turkey rashers; 1 piece fresh fruit

Mid-morning Power Snack

1 small banana

Lunch

50g wafer thin ham, chicken, turkey or beef or 75g low-fat cottage cheese served with a large salad; 1 low-fat yogurt (max. 100 kcal and 5% fat) Ⓥ

Mid-afternoon Power Snack

2 satsumas

Dinner

Fresh Tomato and Basil Pasta (see recipe, page 221) served with a mixed salad Ⓥ

ACTIVITY CHALLENGE

• Walk up and down stairs 4 times consecutively

• Do 4 × 6 reps of tricep dips on the stairs (see Day 5, page 56)

Day Twenty-four

Breakfast
1 blue portion pot/40g unsweetened muesli, topped with 1 chopped apple or pear, served with milk from allowance Ⓥ

Mid-morning Power Snack
1 peach

Lunch
1 thick slice wholegrain bread, toasted, topped with 1 × 70g can sardines in tomato sauce, plus a small salad

Mid-afternoon Power Snack
1 small banana

Dinner
Chicken Dolmades (see recipe, page 157) served with 100g boiled baby new potatoes (with skins) and unlimited fresh vegetables

ACTIVITY CHALLENGE

• Walk briskly for 30 minutes

• Do 10 minutes of toning exercises from this book (see page 255–63) or from a fitness DVD

Day Twenty-five

Breakfast
1 slice wholegrain bread, toasted, spread with savoury sauce, e.g. tomato ketchup, brown sauce or fruity sauce, topped with 2 grilled turkey rashers and 3 grilled tomatoes

Mid-morning Power Snack
8 carrot sticks with 25g low-fat salsa

Lunch
5 pieces any fresh fruit (excluding bananas) Ⓥ

Mid-afternoon Power Snack
½ Rosemary Conley Low Gi Nutrition Bar (eat other half on Day 27)

Dinner
1 × 150g salmon steak, grilled, served with 115g boiled new potatoes (with skins) plus a mixed salad and 1 tbsp low-fat salad dressing

ACTIVITY CHALLENGE

• Do a 40-minute aerobic workout (work out at an aerobics class, to a fitness DVD or on cardio equipment at the gym)

Day Twenty-Six

Breakfast

1 × 100g pot low-fat yogurt (max. 75 kcal and 5% fat) mixed with 1 small sliced banana and 1 yellow portion pot/70g blueberries Ⓥ

Mid-morning Power Snack

1 apple or pear

Lunch

Omelette made with 2 medium eggs and milk from allowance, filled with 25g sliced wafer thin ham, 2 sliced spring onions and chopped mixed peppers, plus a mixed salad

Mid-afternoon Power Snack

2 satsumas

Dinner

Easy Beef Curry (see recipe, page 175) served with 1 blue portion pot/55g (uncooked weight) or 1 red portion pot/144g (cooked weight) boiled basmati rice plus mango chutney and a side salad

ACTIVITY CHALLENGE

• Walk up and down stairs 5 times consecutively

• Do 10 minutes of toning exercises from this book (see pages 255–63) or from a fitness DVD

Day Twenty-seven

Breakfast

1 whole grapefruit or 200g canned grapefruit in natural juice plus 1 slice toasted wholegrain bread spread with 1 tsp jam, honey or marmalade Ⓥ

Mid-morning Power Snack

½ Rosemary Conley Low Gi Nutrition Bar

Lunch

1 × 175g sweet potato baked in its skin and topped with 1 blue portion pot/100g low-fat cottage cheese mixed with 1 tsp chilli sauce, chopped red onion and peppers, plus a small salad Ⓥ

Mid-afternoon Power Snack

2 satsumas

Dinner

Chicken stir-fry: Cut 1 × 115g chicken breast (no skin) into strips and dry-fry with unlimited sliced vegetables. Just before serving add soy sauce to taste plus 1 tbsp sweet chilli dipping sauce to the pan. Serve with 1 blue portion pot/55g (uncooked weight) or 1 red portion pot/144g (cooked weight) boiled basmati rice

Day Twenty-eight

Breakfast
1 slice toasted wholegrain bread topped with
1 scrambled egg and 2 grilled tomatoes Ⓥ

Mid-morning Power Snack
150g strawberries with 1 tsp 0% fat Greek-style
yogurt

Lunch
Assorted salad leaves topped with sliced peppers and
cherry tomatoes and served with 1 blue portion
pot/100g low-fat cottage cheese mixed with 1 blue
portion pot/80g low-fat coleslaw; 1 peach and 100g
strawberries Ⓥ

Mid-afternoon Power Snack
2 satsumas

Dinner
Fillet Steak with Redcurrant
and Thyme Glaze (see recipe,
page 168) served with 115g
boiled new potatoes (with
skins) and unlimited other
vegetables

ACTIVITY CHALLENGE

• Take a 45-minute brisk
walk or bike ride

• Do 10 minutes of toning
exercises from this book
(see pages 255–63) or from
a fitness DVD

Week 4 Shopping List

All meal suggestions and recipes serve one except for Easy Beef Curry, which serves 4 and can be frozen. Otherwise, if preparing meals for more than one person or substituting meals from chapter 11, you will need to amend the shopping list accordingly.

**Store cupboard items
(in addition to Weeks 1 to 3)**
brown or fruity sauce
kaffir lime leaves
lime pickle
medium curry powder
redcurrant jelly
tomato ketchup
vegetable stock powder

Breakfast cereals and bread
1 sliced wholegrain loaf
1 Rosemary Conley Low Gi Nutrition Bar (from box bought in
   Week 2)

Canned foods
1 small can tuna in brine
1 × 70g can sardines in tomato sauce
2 × 400g cans chopped tomatoes
1 small can sweetcorn (25g needed)
vine leaves in brine (2 needed)
sundried tomatoes (2 needed)

Dairy

2.8 litres/5 pints skimmed or semi-skimmed milk

3 eggs (use ones from Week 1)

1 small pot 0% fat Greek yogurt

1 small pot low-fat natural yogurt (max. 75 kcal and 5% fat)

1 small pot virtually fat free fromage frais

1 × 200g pot low-fat cottage cheese

Fresh meat and fish

2 × 150g chicken breasts

1 × 115g chicken breast

450g beef steak

1 × 150g rump steak

1 × 150g salmon steak

25g wafer thin ham

From the chiller cabinet

1 small carton low-fat coleslaw

1 pack turkey rashers (3 rashers needed)

1 Rosemary Conley Ready To Eat Porridge (available from Morrisons or Asda) or use porridge oats from Week 1

Fresh fruit

4 apples or pears

4 small bananas

2 peaches

6 satsumas

1 grapefruit (or 200g canned)

70g blueberries

25g mixed berries

250g strawberries
6 pieces fresh fruit of your choice

Fresh vegetables and salad items
1 pack beansprouts
2 red peppers
2 green peppers
2 yellow peppers
1 pack cherry tomatoes
5 large tomatoes
1 pack carrots
mixed salad leaves
1 cucumber
1 bunch spring onions
3 red onions
1 white onion
extra vegetables of your choice (enough for 2 portions)
330g new potatoes
2 × 175g sweet potatoes (for baking)

Fresh herbs and spices
basil leaves
coriander
mint leaves
thyme
1 garlic bulb

Free Choice Diet Menus plus Extras

Remember, you can choose any breakfast, lunch or dinner on Phase 1 and Phase 2 of the diet. In Phase 2, you can also add a dessert, a high-fat or low-fat treat and an alcoholic drink each day if your calorie allowance permits.

If you still have weight to lose after completing the first four weeks of the diet, then stay on the diet for as long as it takes you to reach your goal. Just select your meals from the following pages – a breakfast, lunch and dinner each day, plus of course your dessert, alcohol and treats if appropriate.

Continue to do the activity challenges at the level recommended in Week 4 of the eating plan. It is vital that you maintain your new, active lifestyle if you want to have a great-looking body at the end of your slimming campaign. Don't forget to use your portion pots to ensure you are eating the correct amounts. At the end of each month, check your daily calorie allowance in the charts on pages 288–91, as you may need to adjust your calorie intake to ensure you maintain a steady rate of weight loss. Alternatively, add in some extra aerobic exercise so that you burn more calories.

Breakfasts

Approx. 200 calories each

cereal breakfasts

* ✱ 1 blue portion pot/40g muesli served with milk from allowance and 1 chopped nectarine or peach Ⓥ
* ✱ 1 yellow portion pot/25g Sultana Bran served with milk from allowance, 1 sliced nectarine or peach, and 1 tbsp 0% fat Greek-style yogurt (e.g. Total 0%) Ⓥ
* ✱ 2 Weetabix served with milk from allowance, 1 tsp sugar and 1 red portion pot/115g raspberries Ⓥ
* ✱ 1 red portion pot/60g All-Bran served with milk from allowance and 1 tsp sugar Ⓥ
* ✱ 1 red portion pot/50g bran flakes served with milk from allowance and 1 tsp sugar Ⓥ
* ✱ 1 blue portion pot/40g muesli topped with 1 chopped apple or pear and served with milk from allowance Ⓥ
* ✱ 1 blue portion pot/40g unsweetened muesli soaked overnight in 1 blue portion pot/80ml unsweetened apple juice and topped with 1 tsp very low fat natural yogurt Ⓥ
* ✱ 1 Weetabix or Shredded Wheat served with milk from allowance, 1 tsp sugar and 1 thinly sliced small banana Ⓥ

continued

* 1 blue portion pot/35g (uncooked weight) porridge oats cooked with water, served with milk from allowance and 1 tsp honey or brown sugar; 1 piece fresh fruit Ⓥ.
* Fruity porridge made with 1 blue portion pot/35g (uncooked weight) porridge oats cooked in water served with milk from allowance and ½ tsp honey or brown sugar, 1 red portion pot/115g raspberries and 25g fresh berries Ⓥ
* 1 pot Rosemary Conley Ready to Eat Porridge plus 1 kiwi fruit Ⓥ
* 1 red portion pot/30g Sugar Puffs mixed with 100g low-fat fruit yogurt (max. 75 kcal and 5% fat) Ⓥ
* 1 red portion pot/30g Sugar Puffs served with 115g canned peaches in natural juice Ⓥ
* 1 red portion pot/40g Special K served with milk from allowance and 115g sliced strawberries Ⓥ
* 1 yellow portion pot/20g Special K mixed with 1 pot low-fat yogurt (max. 100 kcal and 5% fat) Ⓥ
* 1 yellow portion pot/125ml fresh orange juice plus 1 red portion pot/50g bran flakes served with milk from allowance and 1 tsp sugar Ⓥ
* 2 Shredded Wheat served with milk from allowance and 2 tsps sugar plus 1 kiwi fruit Ⓥ
* 1 yellow portion pot/50g muesli served with 1 tsp sugar and milk from allowance Ⓥ

Fruit breakfasts

* ½ melon filled with 1 red portion pot/115g raspberries and topped with 1 pot low-fat yogurt (max. 100 kcal and 5% fat) Ⓥ

* 1 pot low-fat yogurt (max. 75 kcal and 5% fat) mixed with 1 medium sliced banana and 1 red portion pot/115g raspberries or strawberries Ⓥ

* Summer berry smoothie: Blend 100g fresh seasonal berries with 100g virtually fat free fromage frais and milk from allowance; 1 × 35g Rosemary Conley Low Gi Nutrition bar (from www.rosemaryconley.com) Ⓥ

* Fruit salad made with 200g fresh seasonal berries and 1 blue portion pot/80ml unsweetened orange juice, topped with 1 × 150g pot 0% fat Greek-style yogurt Ⓥ

* 1 × 100g pot low-fat yogurt (max. 75 kcal and 5% fat) mixed with 1 tbsp unsweetened muesli and 1 red portion pot/115g raspberries Ⓥ

* 1 small banana, sliced, mixed with 115g sliced strawberries and 1 × 100g pot low-fat yogurt (max. 100 kcal and 5% fat) Ⓥ

* Gi fruit salad: 1 satsuma, broken into segments, 1 chopped pear, 25g seedless grapes and 15g oats. Mix with 1 blue portion pot/80g 0% fat Greek-style yogurt Ⓥ

continued

* 1 × 100g pot low-fat yogurt (max. 75 kcal and 5% fat) mixed with 1 small sliced banana and 1 yellow portion pot/70g blueberries Ⓥ
* 3 prunes and 2 dried apricots, soaked overnight in hot black tea (sweetened with artificial sweetener if desired), topped with 1 blue portion pot/80g low-fat natural yogurt and ½ tsp honey Ⓥ
* 100g canned peaches in natural juice plus 1 × 150g pot low-fat yogurt (max. 150 kcal and 5% fat) Ⓥ
* 4 dried apricots, soaked overnight in hot black tea (sweetened with a little sweetener if required) and a pinch of cinnamon plus 1 × 150g pot low-fat yogurt (max. 150 kcal and 5% fat) Ⓥ
* 150g stewed fruit (cooked with artificial sweetener) plus 1 × 100g pot low-fat yogurt (max. 100 kcal and 5% fat) Ⓥ
* 175g fruit compote (e.g. oranges, grapefruit, peaches, pineapple, pears – all in natural juice) Ⓥ
* 1 whole fresh grapefruit plus 1 × 150g pot low-fat yogurt (max. 150 kcal and 5% fat) Ⓥ
* 5 prunes (in natural juice) plus 1 blue portion pot/80g 0% fat Greek-style yogurt Ⓥ
* 4 pieces any fresh fruit (excluding bananas) Ⓥ
* 2 large bananas Ⓥ
* 1 whole grapefruit or ½ × 400g can grapefruit in natural juice plus 1 slice toasted wholegrain bread spread with 1 tsp jam, marmalade or honey Ⓥ

Cooked breakfasts

* 2 low-fat beef or pork sausages (max. 5% fat) or 4 Quorn sausages, grilled, served with 225g grilled fresh tomatoes or 200g canned tomatoes boiled well and reduced
* 1 slice toasted wholegrain bread topped with 1 yellow portion pot/115g baked beans; 1 piece fresh fruit Ⓥ
* 1 poached or dry-fried egg served with 1 low-fat beef or pork sausage (max. 5% fat) or 1 Quorn sausage, grilled, plus 3 grilled tomatoes and 100g grilled mushrooms Ⓥ
* ½ pink grapefruit, plus 1 medium-sized poached or boiled egg with 1 slice toasted wholegrain bread Ⓥ
* 1 yellow portion pot/125ml unsweetened fruit juice, 1 slice toasted wholegrain bread topped with 1 yellow portion pot/115g baked beans Ⓥ
* 1 slice toasted wholegrain bread spread with savoury sauce, e.g. tomato ketchup, brown sauce or fruity sauce, topped with 2 grilled turkey rashers plus 3 grilled tomatoes
* 1 lean bacon rasher, grilled, served with 100g mushrooms, cooked in stock, 225g canned tomatoes, boiled until reduced (or 4 fresh tomatoes, grilled), plus ½ slice toasted wholegrain bread

continued

* 1 slice toasted wholegrain bread topped with
  1 × 150g can baked beans and 2 grilled
  tomatoes Ⓥ
* 1 poached or dry-fried egg served with 1 grilled lean
  bacon rasher, 2 grilled tomatoes and 115g grilled
  mushrooms
* 1 slice toasted wholegrain bread topped with
  1 scrambled egg and 2 grilled tomatoes Ⓥ
* Turkey rasher sandwich: Spread 1 slice wholegrain
  bread with tomato ketchup, cut in half and make
  into a sandwich with 3 slices grilled turkey rashers;
  1 piece fresh fruit
* 1 poached or dry fried egg served with 2 grilled
  turkey rashers and unlimited grilled tomatoes

Quick and easy breakfasts

* 1 × 35g Rosemary Conley Low GI Nutrition Bar (from www.rosemaryconley.com) plus 2 pieces fresh fruit (e.g. peach, nectarine, apple or kiwi) Ⓥ
* 1 × 35g Rosemary Conley Low Gi Nutrition Bar, any flavour, plus 1 satsuma or clementine and 1 small banana Ⓥ
* 1 small wholegrain roll, cut in half, thinly spread with Philadelphia Extra Light soft cheese, topped with 25g smoked salmon and sprinkled with black pepper
* 1 pot Rosemary Conley Ready to Eat Porridge (from Morrisons or Asda) plus 1 kiwi fruit Ⓥ
* ½ pink grapefruit, 1 medium-sized poached egg served on 1 slice toasted wholegrain bread Ⓥ
* 1 slice toasted wholegrain bread spread with 2 tsps honey, jam or marmalade, plus 1 piece any fresh fruit Ⓥ
* 1 slice wholegrain bread, soaked in 1 beaten egg and milk from allowance, fried with a little spray oil and topped with 1 tsp maple syrup Ⓥ
* 1 slice toasted wholegrain bread spread with 25g Philadelphia Extra Light soft cheese and topped with 1 sliced apple or pear Ⓥ

continued

* 1 small wholemeal roll, cut in half, spread with low-fat dressing of your choice and filled with 50g lean ham plus 2 sliced tomatoes
* 1 small wholemeal roll, spread with Branston pickle or similar, filled with 50g sliced chicken or turkey breast plus 2 sliced tomatoes
* 2 low-fat Scotch pancakes (e.g. Tesco Healthy Living) topped with 2 tsps 0% fat Greek-style yogurt plus 1 red portion pot/115g raspberries or 6 sliced strawberries Ⓥ
* 1 crumpet, toasted, topped with 2 tsps jam or honey and 1 tsp 0% fat Greek-style yogurt Ⓥ
* 1 Müllerlight Corner Healthy Balance yogurt plus 5 sliced strawberries or 10 grapes Ⓥ

Lunches

Approx. 300 calories each

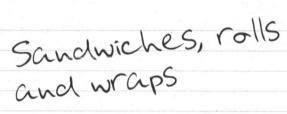

Sandwiches, rolls and wraps

* 2 slices wholegrain bread spread with low-calorie salad dressing and made into a sandwich with 25g wafer thin ham, chicken, beef, turkey or smoked salmon or ¼ blue portion pot/25g low-fat cottage cheese mixed with 1 tbsp canned sweetcorn, plus a small salad Ⓥ
* BLT sandwich: 2 slices wholegrain bread, toasted, 1 slice spread with 1 tsp Hellmann's Extra Light Mayonnaise and the other with tomato ketchup, filled with 25g lean grilled bacon, 1 slice wafer thin chicken, lettuce leaves and sliced tomatoes
* 1 × 50g slice wholegrain baguette, rubbed with a cut garlic clove, toasted, then topped with 1 blue portion pot/80g 0% fat Greek-style yogurt mixed with chopped cucumber, plus sliced tomatoes and a small salad Ⓥ
* Any pre-packed sandwich of your choice made with wholegrain bread (max. 250 kcal and 5% fat), plus a small salad Ⓥ

continued

* 1 small granary baguette filled with 50g diced, cooked beetroot, 50g smoked trout fillets plus watercress or rocket leaves, served with 1 blue portion pot/80g virtually fat-free fromage frais mixed with 1 tsp horseradish sauce, plus a small salad

* 1 small wholegrain roll, cut in half, spread with 25g Philadelphia Extra Light soft cheese and topped with 25g smoked salmon, black pepper plus a small salad

* 1 small wholegrain roll spread with horseradish sauce and topped with 50g wafer thin beef and sliced tomatoes, plus a salad

* 1 small wholegrain roll spread with Philadelphia Extra Light soft cheese and topped with 1 large sliced tomato, fresh basil leaves and black pepper, plus a large salad Ⓥ

* Smoked Mackerel and Horseradish Pâté (see recipe, page 209) served with 2 slices melba toast, plus a salad

* 1 medium wholemeal pitta bread filled with 25g low-fat houmous, shredded lettuce, sliced tomato and cucumber and chopped red pepper, plus a small green salad Ⓥ

* 1 tortilla wrap (max. 200 kcal) spread with 1 tbsp mild tomato salsa and filled with 25g chicken plus salad leaves

continued

* 1 slice toasted wholegrain bread topped with 150g drained canned tuna in brine mixed with 1 tsp low-fat mayonnaise, 1 blue portion pot/80g 0% fat Greek-style yogurt (e.g. Total 0%) and lemon juice. Serve with a small salad
* 1 medium pitta bread filled with shredded lettuce, sliced peppers, spring onions, tomatoes plus 50g canned salmon or low-fat cottage cheese mixed with 1 tbsp sweetcorn Ⓥ
* 1 medium wholemeal pitta bread filled with 1 blue portion pot/75g tomato salsa, plus a handful of rocket, sliced cucumber and 50g sliced, cooked chicken (no skin)
* 1 tortilla wrap (max. 200 kcal) thinly spread with extra light mayonnaise and filled with 50g drained cannned tuna in brine mixed with chopped red onion plus salad leaves
* 1 tortilla wrap (max. 200 kcal) spread with 1 tbsp low-calorie coleslaw and filled with 50g wafer thin pastrami
* 1 tortilla wrap (max. 200 kcal) spread with extra light soft cheese and filled with 25g smoked salmon plus rocket leaves
* 1 tortilla wrap (max. 200 kcal) spread with 1 tsp horseradish sauce and filled with 25g wafer thin beef plus watercress leaves

Salad lunches

* 1 × 150g chicken breast (no skin), grilled, served with a mixed salad tossed in fat-free dressing

* Rice salad: Mix 1 blue portion pot/55g (uncooked weight) or 1 red portion pot/144g (cooked weight) boiled basmati rice with chopped spring onions, diced peppers, 1 tbsp sweetcorn, 1 segmented, peeled orange and 2 tbsps fat-free salad dressing. Serve with a small mixed salad Ⓥ

* Salad Nicoise: Toss 150g boiled baby new potatoes (with skins) with 50g cooked thin green beans, crisp lettuce, sliced radishes, 3 halved cherry tomatoes, 100g drained canned tuna in brine and 5 sliced black grapes in fat-free dressing

* 1 medium mixed salad with fat-free dressing served with 25g wafer thin ham, turkey or chicken; 1 × 35g Rosemary Conley Low Gi Nutrition Bar (from www.rosemaryconley.com) and 1 small banana Ⓥ

* Assorted salad leaves topped with sliced peppers and cherry tomatoes served with 115g low-fat cottage cheese mixed with 75g low-fat coleslaw; 1 peach and 100g strawberries Ⓥ

* Vegetable Quinoa Salad (see recipe, page 225) served with a green salad; 1 × 35g Rosemary Conley Low Fat Nutrition Bar Ⓥ

continued

* 50g wafer thin ham, chicken, turkey or beef or 75g low-fat cottage cheese served with a large salad tossed in fat-free dressing; 1 low-fat yogurt (max. 100 kcal and 5% fat) ⓥ

* Chicken Caesar salad: 1 Little Gem lettuce tossed with chopped cucumber chunks, 115g sliced cooked chicken breast (no skin) mixed with 4 tsps low-fat Caesar dressing (max. 5% fat) and topped with a few Parmesan shavings and home-made garlic croutons (cut 1 × 2cm slice from wholegrain baguette and rub with cut clove of garlic. Cut bread into quarters and slowly toast under a preheated grill until golden brown)

* 1 yellow portion pot/45g (uncooked weight) or 1 red portion pot/110g (cooked weight) cooked pasta shapes cooled then mixed with grilled peppers, 6 halved cherry tomatoes and 50g wafer thin pastrami or drained canned tuna in brine and tossed in fat-free dressing, plus a small mixed salad ⓥ

Soup lunches

* Chilli Bean Soup (see recipe, page 144) served with 1 slice wholegrain bread; 2 satsumas Ⓥ
* Roasted Tomato and Basil Soup (see recipe, page 146) served with 1 small wholegrain baguette; 1 Rosemary Conley Low Fat Belgian Chocolate Mousse
* Broccoli and Potato Soup (see recipe, page 142, plus a small salad Ⓥ
* Smoked Salmon and Corn Chowder (see recipe, page 145) served with 1 slice wholegrain bread, plus a small salad
* Spanish Red Pepper Soup (see recipe, page 147) served with 1 slice wholegrain bread, plus a small salad Ⓥ
* 300g fresh or 400g canned tomato soup (max. 150 kcal and 5% fat), served with 1 slice toasted wholegrain bread and a small salad Ⓥ
* Cannellini Bean Soup (see recipe, page 143), plus a salad; 1 piece fresh fruit
* 1 × 400g can any lentil or vegetable soup (max. 200 kcal) topped with a swirl of low-fat yogurt and served with 1 slice wholegrain bread or small wholegrain roll, plus a salad Ⓥ
* Turkey Vegetable Broth (see recipe, page 149) served with 1 small wholegrain baguette, plus a small salad

Hot lunches

* Baked Cheesy Sweet Potato (see recipe, page 228), plus a small green salad; 1 low-fat yogurt (max. 100 kcal and 5% fat) Ⓥ
* 1 × 100g oven-baked sweet potato topped with ½ blue portion pot/50g low-fat cottage cheese mixed with chopped yellow, green and red peppers. Serve with shredded lettuce and cherry tomatoes; 1 piece fresh fruit Ⓥ
* 1 × 175g sweet potato baked in its skin, topped with 1 blue portion pot/100g low-fat cottage cheese mixed with 1 tsp chilli sauce, chopped red onion and peppers and served with a small salad Ⓥ
* 1 × 175g baked sweet potato topped with 1 yellow portion pot/115g baked beans and served with grilled mushrooms, plus a small salad Ⓥ
* 1 × 175g baked sweet potato topped with one of the following plus small salad with fat-free dressing:
    * ½ blue portion pot/50g low-fat cottage cheese mixed with chopped peppers Ⓥ
    * 50g drained canned tuna in brine mixed with 1 tbsp low-fat salad dressing, 1 tbsp 0% fat Greek-style yogurt and 2 tsps sweetcorn kernels
    * 50g baked beans mixed with ½ tsp curry powder and cooked through

continued

* 1 low-fat beef or pork sausage (max. 5% fat) or
  1 Quorn sausage, grilled, plus 1 yellow portion
  pot/115g baked beans, plus 115g grilled
  mushrooms and 1 slice toasted wholegrain bread Ⓥ

* 1 egg, dry-fried, and 2 grilled turkey rashers served
  with unlimited grilled tomatoes and mushrooms,
  plus a small mixed salad

* Leek, Pea, Smoked Ham and Cheese Pasta (see
  recipe, page 195) served with a salad tossed in fat-
  free dressing

* Omelette made with 2 medium eggs, milk from
  allowance and filled with 25g sliced wafer thin ham,
  2 sliced spring onions and chopped mixed peppers,
  plus a small mixed salad

* Omelette made with 2 medium eggs and filled with
  115g sliced grilled mushrooms and 1 blue portion
  pot/20g grated low-fat Cheddar cheese, plus a small
  salad Ⓥ

* Roasted vegetable pasta: Roughly chop 1 red onion,
  ½ red and green pepper and ½ courgette, drizzle
  with a little balsamic vinegar and roast in the oven
  at 350F, 180C, Gas Mark 4 for 30–35 minutes, or
  until well browned. Combine the roasted vegetables
  with 1 yellow portion pot/45g (uncooked weight) or
  1 red portion pot/110g (cooked weight) cooked
  pasta shapes and some chopped fresh basil. Eat hot
  or cold with a small mixed salad Ⓥ

continued

* 2 low-fat beef or pork sausages (max. 5% fat) or
  2 Quorn sausages, grilled, served on 1 slice toasted
  wholegrain bread with 1 × 200g can tomatoes
  boiled until thick and reduced, plus a small salad Ⓥ
* 1 yellow portion pot/45g (uncooked weight) or 1 red
  portion pot/110g (cooked weight) cooked pasta
  shapes tossed with 50g smoked salmon strips and
  1 yellow portion pot/135g virtually fat free fromage
  frais and chopped fresh dill, served with a green
  salad
* 2 medium eggs, scrambled with ½ small chopped
  red chilli (seeds removed), 3 sliced spring onions and
  chopped coriander. Serve with 1 slice toasted
  wholegrain bread and salad Ⓥ
* 1 green portion pot/170g (cooked weight) or
  1 × 65g block (uncooked weight) egg noodles,
  boiled, tossed with unlimited beansprouts, spring
  onions, peppers, 75g flaked cooked salmon, soy
  sauce and chopped fresh coriander, plus a small
  salad
* Tomato and Basil French Bread Pizza (see recipe,
  page 229) plus a mixed salad Ⓥ
* Quick Basil Noodles (see recipe, page 226) plus a
  mixed salad Ⓥ
* ½ × 410g can Stagg Vegetable Garden Vegetable
  Chilli and 1 small wholegrain roll plus a small
  salad Ⓥ

Quick and easy lunches

* 1 slice toasted wholegrain bread topped with 1 × 70g can sardines in tomato sauce, plus a small salad
* 1 slice toasted wholegrain bread topped with 150g drained canned tuna in brine mixed with 1 tsp low-fat mayonnaise, 1 blue portion pot/80g 0% fat Greek-style yogurt and lemon juice, plus a small salad
* 50g cooked chicken breast (no skin) chopped and mixed with 1 tbsp each low-fat yogurt and mango chutney and served on 2 Dark Rye Ryvita crispbreads, plus a small salad
* 5 pieces any fresh fruit (excluding bananas) Ⓥ
* 2 slices toasted wholegrain bread topped with 1 × 150g can baked beans Ⓥ

Dinners

Approx. 400 calories each

Beef dinners

* Fillet Steak with Redcurrant and Thyme Glaze (see recipe, page 168) served with 115g boiled new potatoes (with skins) and unlimited other vegetables
* Creamy Madeira Beef (see recipe, page 170) served with 1 yellow portion pot/100g mashed sweet potatoes creamed with a little virtually fat free fromage frais plus 115g other vegetables
* Braised Beef with Tomatoes and Thyme (see recipe, page 173) served with 115g boiled new potatoes (with skins) and a selection of other vegetables
* Crispy Steak and Kidney Pie (see recipe, page 167) served with 115g boiled new potatoes (with skins) plus unlimited other vegetables
* Beef Stroganoff (see recipe, page 177) served with 1 blue portion pot/55g (uncooked weight) or 1 red portion pot/144g (cooked weight) boiled basmati rice plus fresh green vegetables
* Beef Masala (see recipe, page 176) served with 1 blue portion pot/55g (uncooked weight) or 1 red portion pot/144g (cooked weight) boiled basmati rice

continued

- 75g roast beef with either 1 low-fat Yorkshire pudding or 75g dry-roasted sweet potatoes plus unlimited green vegetables and a little low-fat gravy
- Beef and Mushroom Skewers (see recipe, page 179) served with 1 blue portion pot/55g (uncooked weight) or 1 red portion pot/144g (cooked weight) boiled basmati rice and a salad tossed in oil-free dressing
- Grilled Steak Verde (see recipe, page 169) plus 75g boiled new potatoes (with skins) and unlimited other vegetables
- Paprika Mince (see recipe, page 180) served with 115g boiled new potatoes (in skins) and steamed green vegetables of your choice
- Thai Beef Stir-Fry (see recipe, page 174) served with 1 blue portion pot/55g (uncooked weight) or 1 red portion pot/144g (cooked weight) boiled basmati rice and green beans
- Easy Beef Curry (see recipe, page 175) served with 1 blue portion pot/55g (uncooked weight) or 1 red portion pot/144g (cooked weight) boiled basmati rice, mango chutney and a side salad
- Boozy Beef with Mushrooms (see recipe, page 171) served with 100g boiled new potatoes (with skins) plus unlimited other vegetables
- Beef and Root Vegetable Stew (see recipe, page 172) served with fresh green vegetables

continued

* Savoury Meatloaf with Caramelised Onion Gravy
  (see recipe, page 181), served with 100g boiled new
  potatoes (with skins) and unlimited fresh vegetables
* Any ready meal (max. 400 kcal and 5% fat)

Lamb dinners

* Lamb Chasseur (see recipe, page 183) served with 100g boiled baby new potatoes (with skins) and 100g other vegetables
* Tunisian Lamb (see recipe, page 187) served with 1 blue portion pot/55g (uncooked weight) or 1 red portion pot/144g (cooked weight) boiled basmati rice
* Spicy Lamb with Sweet Potatoes (see recipe, page 188) served with unlimited fresh vegetables (excluding potatoes)
* Minted Lamb Samosas (see recipe, page 184) (3 samosas per person) served with 1 blue portion pot/55g (uncooked weight) or 1 red portion pot/144g (cooked weight) boiled basmati rice and a small green salad plus 1 tbsp mango chutney
* Fillet of Lamb with Minted Couscous (see recipe, page 185) served with unlimited vegetables (excluding potatoes)
* 115g lamb's liver braised in gravy and sliced onions, served with 115g boiled new potatoes (with skins) and unlimited other vegetables
* Any ready meal (max. 400 kcal and 5% fat)

Pork and gammon dinners

* Pork and Pineapple Kebabs (see recipe, page 191) served with 115g boiled new potatoes (with skins), 1 tsp sweet chilli sauce and 115g green vegetables or a mixed salad tossed in fat-free dressing
* Stir-Fried Pork with Peppers (see recipe, page 190) served with 1 green portion pot/170g (cooked weight) (65g uncooked weight) boiled egg noodles
* Simple Citrus Gammon (see recipe, page 196) served with 115g boiled new potatoes (with skins) and unlimited other vegetables
* Lime and Ginger Stir-Fried Pork (see recipe, page 192) served with 1 blue portion pot/55g (uncooked weight) or 1 red portion pot/144g (cooked weight) boiled basmati rice
* 2 low-fat pork sausages (max. 5% fat) served with Vegetable Fried Rice (see recipe, page 227) served with sauce of your choice
* 2 low-fat beef or pork sausages (max. 5% fat), grilled, served with 1 yellow portion pot/100g mashed sweet potatoes plus unlimited vegetables and low-fat gravy; 1 × Rosemary Conley Low Fat Belgian Chocolate Mousse

continued

* Passionate Pork Casserole (see recipe, page 193) served with 115g boiled baby new potatoes (with skins) and unlimited green vegetables
* Sweet and Sour Pork Slices (see recipe, page 194) served with 115g boiled new potatoes (with skins) and a crisp mixed salad or unlimited fresh vegetables (excluding potatoes)
* Gammon and Pineapple Stir-Fry (see recipe, page 197) served with 1 blue portion pot/55g (uncooked weight) or 1 red portion pot/144g (cooked weight) boiled basmati rice
* Any ready meal (max. 400 kcal and 5% fat)

Chicken, turkey and duck dinners

* Marinated Barbecue Chicken (see recipe, page 160) served with 75g boiled new potatoes (with skins), a little fresh tomato salsa and a small mixed salad tossed in fat-free dressing
* Chicken with Tangerine and Cinnamon (see recipe, page 153) served with 115g boiled new potatoes (with skins) and other seasonal vegetables
* 1 × 175g serving Herby Lemon Roast Chicken (see recipe, page 158) served with 75g dry-roasted sweet potatoes plus 115g fresh vegetables (excluding potatoes) and low-fat gravy
* Chicken with Lime and Ginger (see recipe, page 152) served with 1 blue portion pot/55g (uncooked weight) or 1 red portion pot/144g (cooked weight) boiled basmati rice
* Spicy Chicken Pasta (see recipe, page 163)
* Turkey and Pepper Burgers (see recipe, page 162) served with 1 × 250g (uncooked weight) baked sweet potato, 1 tbsp tomato relish and unlimited salad tossed in fat-free dressing
* Chicken, Leek and Potato Pie (see recipe, page 154) plus unlimited green salad

continued

* Creamy Pineapple Chicken (see recipe, page 161) served with 1 green portion pot/170g (cooked weight) or 65g (uncooked weight) boiled noodles
* Sticky Onion Chicken (see recipe, page 151) served with 1 blue portion pot/55g (uncooked weight) or 1 red portion pot/144g (cooked weight) boiled basmati rice and salad
* Mango and Mushroom Chicken Stir-Fry (see recipe, page 159) served with 1 blue portion pot/55g (uncooked weight) or 1 red portion pot/144g (cooked weight) boiled basmati rice
* 175g chicken breast (no skin), wrapped in foil and cooked under the grill for 15 minutes, turning occasionally to ensure it is thoroughly cooked. Serve with 115g boiled sweet potatoes, unlimited other vegetables of your choice plus a little low-fat gravy
* Chicken Dolmades (see recipe, page 157) served with 100g boiled baby new potatoes (with skins) and unlimited other vegetables
* Quick chicken stir-fry: Cut 1 × 115g chicken breast into strips and dry-fry in non-stick pan with unlimited sliced vegetables (e.g. onions, peppers, carrots and beansprouts); add soy sauce and 1 tbsp sweet chilli dipping sauce to the pan before serving with 1 blue portion pot/55g (uncooked weight) or 1 red portion pot/144g (cooked weight) boiled basmati rice

continued

* Chicken and Mushroom Tortillas (see recipe, page 155) served with unlimited vegetables (excluding potatoes) or a mixed salad
* Fruity Orange Chicken (see recipe, page 156) served with 115g boiled baby new potatoes (with skins) and fresh vegetables
* 1 × 150g chicken breast (no skin), grilled, served with tomato and pepper sauce: dry-fry ½ red onion with ½ each red and green pepper, add small can chopped tomatoes and dash of Worcestershire sauce and season with black pepper. Boil until reduced slightly and add fresh basil if desired. Serve with 1 blue portion pot/55g (uncooked weight) or 1 red portion pot/144g (cooked weight) boiled basmati rice
* Turkey and Bacon Hotpot (see recipe, page 164) served with unlimited vegetables (excluding potatoes)
* Roman saltimbocca: Wrap 1 × 125g skinned chicken or turkey breast steak in 1 thin slice Parma ham and grill for about 5–8 minutes each side until browned and the chicken is cooked through. Cook 1 blue portion pot/50g (uncooked weight) couscous according to instructions and stir in some chopped chilli, spring onion and herbs. Serve with the chicken and griddled courgettes, peppers and aubergines

continued

* 115g roast chicken or turkey (no skin), served with
  115g dry-roasted sweet potatoes, 75g dry-roast
  parsnips plus unlimited other vegetables and a little
  low-fat gravy
* Pan-Fried Duck with Black Bean Sauce (see recipe,
  page 165) served with 1 blue portion pot/55g
  (uncooked weight) or 1 red portion pot/144g
  (cooked weight) boiled basmati rice and unlimited
  steamed pak choi
* 1 × 425g pack Rosemary Conley's Sweet Chilli and
  Chicken Noodles seved with steamed green
  vegetables
* Any ready meal (max. 400 kcal and 5% fat)

Fish and seafood dinners

* 1 × 150g tuna steak sprinkled with black pepper and lime juice, grilled, served with 1 blue portion pot/55g (uncooked weight) or 1 red portion pot/144g (cooked weight) basmati rice, plus stir-fry vegetables (peppers, beansprouts, ½ red onion, coarsely grated carrot) dry-fried with a little soy sauce
* Baked Parma Ham Cod with Saffron Couscous (see recipe, page 201) served with 115g broccoli and 115g mangetout
* Seafood Chowder (see recipe, page 148) served with 1 small wholegrain baguette, plus a small salad
* Spiced Tomato Baked Cod (see recipe, page 198) served with 1 blue portion pot/55g (uncooked weight) or 1 red portion pot/144g (cooked weight) boiled basmati rice, plus seasonal vegetables or salad tossed in fat-free dressing
* Tuna and Tomato Pasta (see recipe, page 204) served with a mixed salad; plus 1 Rosemary Conley Low Fat Belgian Chocolate Mousse
* King Prawn Risotto (see recipe, page 208) served with unlimited salad or steamed vegetables (excluding potatoes)

continued

- ✳ Marinated Griddled Tuna (see recipe, page 203) served with 1 blue portion pot/55g (uncooked weight) or 1 red portion pot/144g (cooked weight) boiled basmati rice and salad or vegetables (excluding potatoes) of your choice
- ✳ Ginger Baked Smoked Salmon (see recipe, page 205) served with 200g boiled new potatoes (with skins), plus unlimited other vegetables, cherry tomatoes and a little 0% Greek-style yogurt
- ✳ Roast Smoked Cod with Cheese and Chive Sauce (see recipe, page 199) served with 80g boiled new potatoes (with skins) and a selection of other vegetables
- ✳ Smoky Prawn Stir-Fry (see recipe, page 200) served with 1 blue portion pot/55g (uncooked weight) or 1 red portion pot/144g (cooked weight) boiled basmati rice
- ✳ Pan-Fried Sea Bass with Spinach and Mushrooms (see recipe, page 202) served with 1 yellow portion pot/100g mashed sweet potatoes and unlimited other vegetables of your choice
- ✳ 1 × 175g tuna steak, grilled, served with any low-fat relish or tomato salsa, 115g boiled new potatoes (with skins) and unlimited green vegetables
- ✳ 1 × 175g salmon steak, grilled or steamed, served with 115g boiled new potatoes (with skins) and unlimited green vegetables

continued

* 1 × 150g salmon steak, grilled or steamed, served with 115g boiled new potatoes (with skins) and unlimited green vegetables
* 200g steamed white fish served with 115g boiled new potatoes (with skins) and unlimited vegetables of your choice plus low-fat parsley sauce
* 1 × 175g baked sweet potato topped with 100g drained canned tuna in brine, drained and mixed with 4 tsps low-fat salad dressing, 25g canned sweetcorn and 2 tsps 0% fat Greek-style yogurt. Serve with a large salad tossed in fat-free dressing
* Marinated Monkfish with Fragrant Rice (see recipe, page 207) served with unlimited vegetables (excluding potatoes)
* Thai Salmon Steaks (see recipe, page 306) served with a mixed salad tossed in fat-free dressing and 50g boiled baby new potatoes (with skins)
* 1 × 425g pack Rosemary Conley's King Prawn and Ginger with Basmati Egg Rice, plus salad
* Any ready meal (max. 400 kcal and 5% fat)

Vegetarian dinners

* Fresh Tomato and Basil Pasta (see recipe, page 221) served with mixed salad leaves tossed in fat-free dressing Ⓥ
* Tofu Noodle Stir-Fry (see recipe, page 211) served with unlimited seasonal vegetables (excluding potatoes) Ⓥ
* Apricot and Vegetable Kebabs with Sweet Chilli Dipping Sauce (see recipe, page 213) served with 1 blue portion pot/55g (uncooked weight) or 1 red portion pot/144g (cooked weight) boiled basmati rice, plus a mixed salad Ⓥ
* Quorn Fajitas (see recipe, page 215) served with unlimited salad tossed in fat-free dressing Ⓥ
* Pasta Arrabiata (see recipe, page 224) served with a mixed salad tossed in fat-free dressing Ⓥ
* Courgette Pasta Bake (see recipe, page 219) served with fresh vegetables (excluding potatoes) or salad tossed in oil-free dressing; 115g fresh fruit salad and 1 tbsp 0% fat Greek-style yogurt Ⓥ
* Parsnip and Pistachio Cutlets (see recipe, page 210) served with tomato salsa and a large green salad. 115g fresh fruit salad and 1 tbsp 0% fat Greek-style yogurt Ⓥ

continued

* Citrus Tofu Stir-Fry with Noodles (see recipe, page 212) served with a crisp green salad; 1 × 150g low-fat yogurt (max. 100 kcal and 5 % fat) Ⓥ
* Pasta with Creamy Tomato Pesto (see recipe, page 220) served with mixed salad tossed in fat-free dressing; 100g 0 % fat Greek-style yogurt plus ½ tsp runny honey Ⓥ
* Creamy Vegetable Tagliatelle (see recipe, page 223) served with a large mixed salad Ⓥ
* Red pepper tortilla: Spray a hot pan with a little low-calorie cooking spray (e.g. Fry Light). Add 200g cooked diced potato, 1 diced red pepper, 1 crushed garlic clove and cook until soft. Add 2 medium beaten eggs, seasoning to taste and chopped parsley. Cook gently until set underneath, then pop under a hot grill to brown the top. Serve in wedges with unlimited green vegetables or salad in fat-free dressing Ⓥ
* Vegetable Pasta Stir-Fry (see recipe, page 222) served with a small green salad tossed in fat-free dressing; 1 × 150g low-fat (max. 75 kcal and 5 % fat) yogurt Ⓥ
* ½ × 410g can Stagg Vegetable Garden Vegetable Chilli served with 1 blue portion pot/55g (uncooked weight) or 1 red portion pot/144g (cooked weight) boiled basmati rice, plus a mixed salad Ⓥ

continued

* Pasta bake: Roast red onion wedges and chunks of aubergine, red pepper and courgette in a little spray oil on a baking tray in a medium oven until soft. When cooked, place the vegetables in an ovenproof dish and add 200g canned tomatoes and seasoning to taste. Cook in the oven for 10 minutes, then add 1 yellow portion pot/45g (uncooked weight) or 1 red portion pot/110g (cooked weight) boiled pasta shapes and bake in the oven for 5–10 minutes. Sprinkle with 2 tsps Parmesan cheese and serve with a small side salad Ⓥ

* Tomato and mushroom pasta: Dry-fry 175g sliced mushrooms lightly with ½ chopped onion and 1 crushed garlic clove. Stir in 200g can chopped tomatoes plus black pepper and chopped fresh basil. Meanwhile, cook 100g (uncooked weight) tagliatelle and combine with the tomato and mushroom mixture. Serve with steamed vegetables or salad Ⓥ

* Okra and Chickpea Stew (see recipe, page 216) served with 1 blue portion pot/55g (uncooked weight) or 1 red portion pot/144g (cooked weight) boiled basmati rice and a small salad Ⓥ

* Potato, Spinach and Cheese Bake (see recipe, page 217) served with steamed broccoli or peas and sweetcorn Ⓥ

continued

* Beans in Red Wine (see recipe, page 218) served with unlimited fresh vegetables Ⓥ
* Stuffed pepper: Dry-fry 1 chopped onion, 1 crushed garlic clove and 1 chopped carrot in a non-stick frying pan. Add 5 chopped mushrooms, 75g Quorn mince and 200g canned chopped tomatoes. Cook for 10 minutes. Meanwhile, split a yellow or red pepper in half, fill with the mixture and sprinkle with 1 tbsp half-fat grated Cheddar cheese. Place on a non-stick baking tray and bake in a preheated oven at 350F, 180C, Gas Mark 4 for 15 minutes. Serve with salad and 1 red portion pot/80g (uncooked weight) or 1 green portion pot/176g (cooked weight) boiled pasta shapes Ⓥ
* 1 red portion pot/80g (uncooked weight) or 1 green portion pot/176g (cooked weight) boiled pasta shapes mixed with ½ jar (approx. 200g) ready-made tomato and basil pasta sauce and heat through. Serve with chopped fresh basil leaves and a sprinkling of Parmesan shavings plus a large green salad Ⓥ
* 1 small low-fat pizza (max. 350 kcal and 5% fat) served with a large mixed salad tossed in fat-free dressing Ⓥ
* Any ready meal (max. 400 kcal and 5% fat) Ⓥ

Power snacks

Approx. 50 kcal each. Select two per day

The following Power Snacks are slow-releasing energy foods that will help sustain your blood sugar levels until your next meal. Ideally, eat one mid-morning and one mid-afternoon.

Fresh fruit
* 2 kiwi fruits
* 1 small or ½ large banana
* 1 medium pear
* 1 medium peach
* 1 medium apple
* 1 medium nectarine
* 1 medium orange
* 1 whole papaya
* 2 satsumas
* 2 fresh figs
* 2 clementines
* 3 plums
* 4 fresh apricots
* 100g pineapple
* 75g seedless grapes
* 100g mango
* 100g cherries
* 1 whole grapefruit
* 150g strawberries or raspberries plus 1 tsp 0% fat Greek-style yogurt

Dried fruit

* 2 dried apricots
* 1 dried fig
* 20g sultanas

Vegetables

* 8 cherry tomatoes
* 150g mixed salad with 1 tsp fat-free dressing
* 8 carrot sticks with 25g low-fat salsa
* 3 celery sticks with 25g low-fat cottage cheese mixed with black pepper and chopped red onion
* 200g mixed salad

Other power snacks

* 15g toasted muesli served with milk from allowance and a little low-calorie sugar substitute Ⓥ
* 1 × 100g pot 0.1% fat Actimel probiotic yogurt drink, any flavour, plus 1 satsuma or clementine Ⓥ
* ½ × 35g Rosemary Conley Low Gi Nutrition Bar Ⓥ
* 1 mini pitta bread with 15g low-fat houmous Ⓥ
* 1 Ryvita Dark Rye crispbread spread with 15g low-fat houmous Ⓥ
* 1 Ryvita Dark Rye crispbread spread with 50g low-fat salsa Ⓥ

Desserts

Under 100 kcal

* Pineapple and Raspberry Crème (see recipe, page 231) 67 kcal
* Honey and Ginger Oranges (see recipe, page 230) 97 kcal
* Rocky Road (see recipe, page 230) 75 kcal
* 2 mini meringues topped with 50g raspberries and 1 tbsp 0% fat Greek-style yogurt 65 kcal
* 1 meringue basket topped with 50g raspberries and 1 tsp 0% fat Greek-style yogurt 80 kcal
* 1 meringue basket topped with 2 tsps 0% fat Greek-style yogurt and 1 chopped kiwi fruit 90 kcal
* 1 Mr Kipling Delightful Apple Slice 91 kcal
* 1 Asda Good For You Chocolate Slice 95 kcal
* 1 Sainsbury's Lemon Cake Slice 97 kcal
* 1 pot Tesco Healthy Living Lemon Cheesecake Yogurt 90 kcal
* 1 × ⅛ slice Soreen Lincolnshire Plum Fruit Loaf 65 kcal
* 1 × 120g pot Del Monte Fruitini Fruit Pieces in Juice 71 kcal
* 1 pot Hartley's Low Sugar Jelly plus 1 piece any fresh fruit 60 kcal
* Chocolate Banana Fool (see recipe, page 234) 92 kcal

Under 125 kcal

✱ Pot Au Chocolat (see recipe, page 232) 117 kcal

✱ 1 pot Rosemary Conley Low Fat Strawberry Mousse 114 kcal

✱ 150g fresh fruit salad plus 1 tsp low-fat yogurt 100 kcal

✱ 1 × 95g pot Müllerlight Fruit Corner Snack Size Strawberry flavour 108 kcal

✱ 1 × 150g pot Ambrosia Low Fat Custard 105 kcal

✱ 2 mini meringues topped with ½ pot Rosemary Conley Low Fat Strawberry Mousse and 50g sliced strawberries 105 kcal

✱ 1 Rosemary Conley Low Fat Belgian Chocolate Mousse 122 kcal

Under 150 kcal

✱ Raspberry Panna Cotta (see recipe, page 233) 129 kcal

✱ 1 Sainsbury's Be Good To Yourself Strawberry Trifle 135 kcal

✱ Sparkling Fresh Fruit Salad (see recipe, page 235) 149 kcal

✱ 1 Sainsbury's Be Good To Yourself Chocolate Sponge Pudding 137 kcal

Treats

Choose one a day if your calorie allowance permits. Remember, you can save up your treats over seven days for a special occasion.

High-fat treats for under 100 kcal

Crisps
* 10 Pringles Lights Sour Cream & Onion flavour 99 kcal
* 25g Jacobs Original Twiglets 97 kcal
* 1 × 21g bag Golden Wonder Golden Lights Sour Cream & Onion flavour 94 kcal
* 1 × 22g bag Walkers French Fries 94 kcal
* 1 × 18g bag Skips Prawn Cocktail 89 kcal
* 1 × 24g bag Kettle Crispy Bakes Mild Cheese with Sweet Onion 91 kcal
* 1 × 25g bag Walkers Squares Ready Salted 94 kcal

Cereal bars and cakes
* 1 Tesco Crazy Caramel Treat Size Cake Bar 95 kcal
* 1 Cadbury Highlights Toffee Flavour Cake Bar 95 kcal
* 1 Mr Kipling Delightful Chocolate Cake Slice 95 kcal
* 1 Harvest Chewee White Choc Chip Cereal Bar 94 kcal
* 1 Kellogg's Special K Bar 90 kcal

Biscuits

* 1 McVities Boasters Belgian Chocolate & Hazelnut flavour 91 kcal
* 3 Cadbury Milk Chocolate Fingers 90 kcal
* 1 McVities Hob Nob 92 kcal
* 3 Rombouts Café Biscuits 92 kcal
* 1 Fox's Golden Crunch Creams 75 kcal
* 2 Jaffa Cakes 88 kcal
* 1 McVities Light Milk Chocolate Digestive 78 kcal
* 1 Tesco All Butter Traditional Scottish Shortbread Finger 90 kcal
* 4 Cadbury Snaps (any flavour) 80 kcal

Sweets and chocolate

* 1 mini bag Nestlé Milkybar Buttons 87 kcal
* 1 Cadbury Dairy Milk Less than 99 kcal bar 95 kcal
* 1 Boots Shapers Crispy Caramel Bar 99 kcal
* 1 × 20g fun size bag M & Ms 98 kcal
* 1 Thorntons Continental Chocolate 70 kcal
* 1 fun size Mars Bar 88 kcal
* 2 segments Terry's Chocolate Orange 90 kcal
* 1 Tesco Value Choc Ice 95 kcal
* 1 Ferrero Rocher 75 kcal

Alcoholic drinks

All these alcoholic drinks are under 100 calories. Use slimline mixers and diet drinks with spirits to keep the calories down.

Beer
* 300ml/½ pint bitter 91 kcal
* 300ml/½ pint lager 82 kcal

Brandy and liqueurs
* 1 × 25ml measure brandy 50 kcal
* 1 × 25ml measure Southern Comfort 81 kcal
* 1 × 25ml measure Tia Maria 75 kcal

Spirits
* 1 × 25ml measure Bacardi 56 kcal
* 1 × 275ml bottle Diet Bacardi Breezer 96 kcal
* 1 × 25ml measure gin 50 kcal
* 1 × 25ml measure vodka 50 kcal
* 1 × 25ml measure whisky 50 kcal

Vermouth

* 1 × 50ml measure Martini Rosso 70 kcal
* 1 × 50ml measure Martini Extra Dry 48 kcal

Wine and fortified wine

* 1 × 125ml glass Champagne 95 kcal
* 1 × 125ml glass dry white wine 83 kcal
* 1 × 125ml glass medium white wine 93 kcal
* 1 × 125ml glass red wine 85 kcal
* 1 × 125ml glass medium rosé wine 89 kcal
* 1 × 50ml measure port 79 kcal
* 1 × 50ml measure sweet sherry 68 kcal
* 1 × 50ml measure dry sherry 58 kcal

Remember – use your yellow portion pot (125ml) to measure wine

Recipes

All preparation and cooking times are approximate

Ⓥ means suitable for vegetarians

❄ means suitable for home freezing

Soups

Broccoli and Potato Soup Ⓥ ❄

SERVES 4
PER SERVING
242 CALORIES
10G FAT
PREP TIME 10 MINUTES
COOK TIME 20 MINUTES

4 long shallots, sliced
115g baby new potatoes, chopped
2 garlic cloves, crushed
1 tsp chopped fresh rosemary
1.2 litres vegetable stock
225g broccoli florets
2 tbsps chopped fresh parsley
salt and freshly ground black pepper

for the blue cheese croutons
40g French bread, cut into 4 thin slices
50g Gorgonzola cheese

1 Place the shallots, potatoes, garlic and rosemary in a large
   saucepan. Pour in the vegetable stock and bring to the boil.
   Simmer gently until the potatoes are cooked.
2 Add the broccoli and parsley and continue cooking until the
   broccoli is tender. Pour into a liquidiser and blend until
   smooth.

3 Return the soup to the saucepan to reheat and add more
   seasoning if required.
4 To make the croutons, lightly toast the
   French bread on both sides under a
   medium grill. Spread with the
   Gorgonzola.
5 Pour the soup into warmed bowls and
   place 2 croutons on top of each one.

Tip

For a creamy soup, stir in 1 tbsp virtually fat free fromage frais just before serving

Cannellini Bean Soup

SERVES 4
PER SERVING
243 CALORIES
6G FAT
PREP TIME 15 MINUTES
COOK TIME 1 HOUR

50g white beans (cannellini or haricot), soaked overnight
4 rashers smoked lean back bacon, cut into strips
4 small shallots, finely sliced
2 garlic cloves, crushed
4 large carrots, diced
1 large celery stick, chopped
2 × 400g cans chopped tomatoes
2 tbsps small pasta shapes
2 tsps chopped fresh oregano
2–3 tsps vegetable stock bouillon powder
4 outer leaves of dark savoy cabbage, finely shredded
freshly ground black pepper

1 Rinse the beans well and place in a large saucepan with the bacon, shallots, garlic, carrots and celery. Cover with water and bring to the boil. Reduce the heat and simmer gently for 30 minutes, topping up with water as required.

2 Add the tomatoes, pasta shapes and oregano. Taste the soup and add sufficient stock powder, adjusting the consistency with more water. Continue to simmer for a further 25 minutes until the beans are soft.

3 Just before serving, add the shredded cabbage and stir it in to wilt. Season well with black pepper and serve hot.

Chilli Bean Soup Ⓥ ❄

SERVES 4
PER SERVING
163 CALORIES
2.7G FAT
PREP TIME 10 MINUTES
COOK TIME 25 MINUTES

1 medium red onion, finely chopped
1 small red chilli, sliced
1 × 200g can chickpeas, drained and rinsed
1 × 200g can red kidney beans, drained and rinsed
1 × 400g can chopped tomatoes
600ml/1 pint vegetable stock
1 tbsp tomato purée
2 tsps chopped fresh oregano
salt and freshly ground black pepper

Tip

For a thick, creamy soup, liquidise in batches and finish with a little semi-skimmed milk

1 Heat a non-stick wok or frying pan. Add the onion and chilli and dry-fry for 4–5 minutes.
2 Transfer to a saucepan and add the remaining ingredients. Simmer gently for 20 minutes. Season to taste with salt and pepper before serving.

Tip

For a milder soup, stir in a little 0% fat Greek-style yogurt before serving

Smoked Salmon and Corn Chowder

SERVES 4
PER SERVING
209 CALORIES
2.4G FAT
PREP TIME 10 MINUTES
COOK TIME 20 MINUTES

2 onions, sliced
2 garlic cloves, crushed
600ml/1 pint vegetable stock
2 tbsps plain flour
600ml/1 pint skimmed milk
225g frozen sweetcorn
225g new potatoes, diced
pinch of dried chilli flakes
115g smoked salmon, chopped
2 tbsps chopped fresh parsley
salt and freshly ground black pepper
low-fat fromage frais, to serve

1 Heat a large non-stick pan, add the onions and garlic and dry-fry for 1–2 minutes until soft.
2 Add 3 tbsps of vegetable stock then sprinkle the flour over and mix in. Cook for 1 minute then stir in the remaining stock and the skimmed milk. Add the sweetcorn, new potatoes and chilli flakes, bring to a gentle simmer and cook until the potatoes are soft.
3 Season to taste with salt and freshly ground black pepper. Just before serving stir in the smoked salmon and chopped parsley.
4 Swirl a little fromage frais on top before serving.

Tip

Add the salmon just before serving as it will soon break up if allowed to simmer

Roasted Tomato and Basil Soup Ⓥ ❄

SERVES 4
PER SERVING
49 CALORIES
1.1G FAT
PREP TIME 10 MINUTES
COOK TIME 45 MINUTES

1kg ripe tomatoes
3 garlic cloves, left whole
600ml/1 pint vegetable stock
handful of basil leaves
salt and freshly ground black pepper

Tip

For a spicy soup, stir in 1 tbsp grated fresh horseradish

1 Preheat the oven to 200C, 400F, Gas Mark 6.
2 Place the tomatoes and garlic cloves in a roasting tin. Season with salt and pepper and bake in the oven for 35 minutes until roasted.
3 Remove the tomatoes from the oven and spoon batches into a food processor or liquidiser. Blend until smooth, adding some of the vegetable stock and basil leaves to each batch.
4 Pass the soup through a sieve into a saucepan and add the remaining vegetable stock. Heat through and season to taste with salt and black pepper. Serve hot or cold.

Spanish Red Pepper Soup ⓥ

SERVES 2
PER SERVING
148 CALORIES
2G FAT
PREP TIME 10 MINUTES
COOK TIME 20 MINUTES

4 long shallots, sliced
1 tsp paprika
2 garlic cloves, crushed
2 red peppers, seeded and diced
1 × 175g can sweetcorn, drained
pinch of dried chilli flakes
600ml/1 pint vegetable stock
1 × 400g can chopped tomatoes
115g new potatoes, chopped
salt and freshly ground black pepper
2 tbsps chopped fresh chives, to garnish

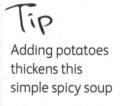

Tip
Adding potatoes thickens this simple spicy soup

1 Heat a large non-stick pan, add the shallots, paprika and garlic and dry-fry for 2–3 minutes. Add the peppers, sweetcorn and chilli flakes and stir in the stock and tomatoes.

2 Bring to the boil, then reduce the heat to a gentle simmer. Add the potatoes and simmer until cooked.

3 Adjust the seasoning and garnish with the chives.

Seafood Chowder

SERVES 4
PER SERVING
225 CALORIES
1.2G FAT
PREP TIME 40 MINUTES
COOK TIME 25 MINUTES

2 onions, finely chopped
2 garlic cloves, crushed
600ml/1 pint vegetable stock
2 tbsps plain flour
1 × 400g can chopped tomatoes
1 small red chilli, seeded and finely chopped
300ml/½ pint tomato passata
450g ready to eat seafood selection
1 tbsp chopped fresh parsley
1 tbsp chopped fresh chives
2 tbsps virtually fat free fromage frais
salt and freshly ground black pepper

Tip

For an extra special touch when entertaining, serve with a thin slice of toasted French bread topped with grated low-fat cheese (adds approx. 60 calories per serving

1 Heat a large, non-stick saucepan, add the onions and dry-fry until soft.
2 Add the garlic and 3 tbsps of stock. Sprinkle the flour over and beat well with a wooden spoon. Cook for 1 minute in order to 'cook out' the flour, then gradually stir in the remaining stock.
3 Add the chopped tomatoes, chilli and tomato passata and simmer gently for 10–15 minutes.
4 Stir in the seafood and herbs and remove the pan from the heat. Add the fromage frais and season to taste with salt and black pepper.
5 Ladle into bowls and serve.

Turkey Vegetable Broth

SERVES 4
PER SERVING
106 CALORIES
1.2G FAT
PREP TIME 10 MINUTES
COOK TIME 25 MINUTES

2 × 125g turkey steaks, cut into thin strips
4 baby leeks, sliced
115g baby carrots, cut in half
2 small courgettes, thinly sliced
1.2 litres/2 pints chicken stock
1 × 400g can chopped tomatoes
1 tbsp chopped fresh herbs (parsley, thyme, oregano)
30g pearl barley
salt and freshly ground black pepper

1 Heat a large, non-stick pan, add the turkey steaks and leeks and dry-fry for 2–3 minutes.
2 Add the remaining ingredients and bring to the boil. Reduce the heat and simmer gently for 20 minutes or until the pearl barley has split and is soft.
3 Adjust the seasoning and serve.

Tip

This soup benefits from being made in advance to allow the flavours to fully develop

Chicken, turkey and duck

Sticky Onion Chicken ✳

SERVES 1
PER SERVING
252 CALORIES
3.7G FAT
PREP TIME 10 MINUTES
MARINATING TIME 1 HOUR
COOK TIME 25–30 MINUTES

1 × 175g skinless chicken breast
salt and freshly ground black pepper

for the marinade
2 tsps sweet chilli sauce
2 tsps runny honey
1 × 1cm piece ginger, peeled and chopped
½ small red onion, finely chopped
juice of ½ lime

> **Tip**
>
> Leave the chicken to marinate overnight in the refrigerator for maximum flavour

1 Season the chicken breast with salt and black pepper and place in the bottom of an ovenproof dish.
2 Combine the marinade ingredients in a mixing bowl. Pour the marinade over the chicken and leave to marinate for at least 1 hour.
3 Preheat the oven to 200C, 400F, Gas Mark 6.
4 Place the chicken, with the marinade, in the oven and bake for 25–30 minutes until fully cooked.
5 Serve straight from the oven.

Chicken with Lime and Ginger

SERVES 1
PER SERVING
240 CALORIES
5G FAT
PREP TIME 10 MINUTES
COOK TIME 20 MINUTES

1 × 150g skinless chicken breast
1 small leek, finely chopped
1 small garlic clove, crushed
pinch of ground ginger
pinch of ground cumin
¼ tsp lemongrass paste
40ml chicken stock
zest and juice of 1 lime
50g Philadelphia Extra Light soft cheese
salt and freshly ground black pepper
1 tsp chopped fresh coriander, to garnish

Tip

For a variation you can use thinly cut turkey breast or pork escalope instead of chicken

1   Cut the chicken breast into thin strips and season with salt and black pepper.
2   Heat a non-stick pan. Add the chicken and cook until lightly browned. Add the, leek, garlic, ginger, cumin and lemongrass paste and continue to cook over a low heat for 2 minutes.
3   Add the chicken stock and the lime zest and juice and bring to a gentle simmer.
4   Fold in the soft cheese and bring back to the boil.
5   Just before serving sprinkle with the coriander.

Chicken with Tangerine and Cinnamon

SERVES 4
PER SERVING
263 CALORIES
4.4G FAT
PREP TIME 15 MINUTES
COOK TIME 35 MINUTES

4 × 150g skinless chicken breasts
4 tangerines
300ml/½ pint fresh apple juice
2 garlic cloves, crushed
2 cinnamon sticks
1 tbsp fresh thyme
1 tbsp plum sauce
2 tsps sweet grain mustard
150ml/¼ pint chicken stock
2 tbsps tomato purée
sea salt and freshly ground black pepper

Tip

For a spicy addition spread the chicken with a little Dijon mustard before pouring the sauce over

1 Preheat the oven to 170C, 325F, Gas Mark 3. Preheat a non-stick frying pan.
2 Season the chicken breasts on both sides with salt and black pepper. Add to the pan and brown on both sides. Transfer to an ovenproof dish.
3 Cut the tangerines in half and squeeze the juice over the chicken, dropping the shells onto the chicken.
4 Mix together the remaining ingredients and pour over the chicken. Cover with a lid or foil and bake in the oven for 30 minutes until the chicken is fully cooked.

Chicken, Leek and Potato Pie ❄

SERVES 4
PER SERVING
408 CALORIES
6.6G FAT
PREP TIME 20 MINUTES
COOK TIME 35 MINUTES

4 × 150g skinned and boned chicken breasts
4 leeks, finely chopped
2 garlic cloves, crushed
1 tbsp chopped fresh basil
2 × 400g cans chopped tomatoes
1 tbsp tomato purée
salt and freshly ground black pepper

for the topping
675g potatoes, peeled and chopped
2 tbsps semi-skimmed milk
50g low-fat mature Cheddar cheese, grated
salt and freshly ground black pepper

Tip

You can substitute turkey or pork for the chicken if you prefer

1 Preheat the oven to 190C, 375F, Gas Mark 5.
2 Cook the potatoes in a pan of boiling water until softened.
3 Meanwhile, preheat a non-stick frying pan. Cut the chicken into bite-sized pieces.
4 Add the chopped chicken and leeks to the pan and dry-fry for 3–4 minutes. Season with salt and black pepper.
5 Add the garlic, basil, tomatoes and tomato purée and allow to simmer gently for 10 minutes.

6 Drain the potatoes. Mash well, adding the milk and half the cheese, and season with salt and black pepper.
7 Spoon the chicken mixture into an ovenproof dish, top with the mashed potatoes and sprinkle with the remaining cheese.
8 Bake in the oven for 25 minutes until golden brown.

Chicken and Mushroom Tortillas ❄

SERVES 4
PER SERVING
372 CALORIES
3.5G FAT
PREP TIME 10 MINUTES
COOK TIME 30 MINUTES

4 × 100g skinless chicken breasts
1 red onion, finely chopped
1 garlic clove, crushed
115g chestnut mushrooms
400g Philadelphia Extra Light soft cheese
1 tsp vegetable stock powder
1 tbsp Dijon mustard
1 tbsp chopped fresh dill
4 small flour tortillas
salt and freshly ground black pepper

1 Preheat the oven to 200C, 400F, Gas Mark 6.
2 Heat a large, non-stick frying pan, dry-fry the chicken breasts, onion and garlic for 4–5 minutes, seasoning with salt and black pepper.

3 Add the mushrooms and continue cooking for 1–2 minutes.

4 Stir in the soft cheese, stock powder, mustard and dill and simmer gently to allow the sauce to thicken. Remove from the heat and allow to cool slightly.

5 Fill each tortilla with the chicken mix and roll up. Place in an ovenproof dish and then in the oven for 15–20 minutes to reheat.

Tip

These tasty tortillas freeze well. Leave to defrost in the refrigerator overnight before reheating

Fruity Orange Chicken ✸

SERVES 4
PER SERVING
263 CALORIES
5.4G FAT
PREP TIME 10 MINUTES
COOK TIME 35 MINUTES

4 × 160g skinless chicken breasts, cut into chunks
1 large onion, sliced
2 garlic cloves, crushed
1 tbsp plain flour
300ml/½ pint chicken stock
1 × 400g can chopped tomatoes
150ml/¼ pint orange juice
1 orange, sliced
1 tbsp chopped fresh coriander
salt and freshly ground black pepper

1 Heat a large, non-stick pan, add the chicken, onion and garlic and dry-fry until the chicken is sealed and the onion is soft.
2 Stir in the flour and cook for 1 minute before gradually stirring in the chicken stock.
3 Add the chopped tomatoes, orange juice and orange slices. Cover and simmer for 25 minutes.
4 Just before serving, mix in the coriander and season to taste with salt and pepper. Serve hot.

Tip

Adding the coriander just before serving keeps its vibrant colour and aromatic flavour

Chicken Dolmades ❄

SERVES 1
PER SERVING
224 CALORIES
8.1G FAT
PREP TIME 15 MINUTES
COOK TIME 20 MINUTES

2 sundried tomatoes
1 × 150g skinless chicken breast
1 tbsp 0% fat Greek yogurt
½ garlic clove, crushed
1 tsp chopped fresh mint
2 vine leaves in brine
salt and freshly ground black pepper

Tip

These minty chicken breasts are also great sliced cold with salad

1 Preheat the oven to 200C, 400F, Gas Mark 6.
2 Place the sundried tomatoes in a small bowl and cover with boiling water. Leave to soak while preparing the chicken.

3 Place the chicken breast on a chopping board and slice across the centre, making a pocket in the breast.
4 Mix together the yogurt, garlic and mint and season with salt and black pepper.
5 Drain the soaked tomatoes. Spoon the tomatoes and half the yogurt mixture inside the breast.
6 Season the chicken breast on both sides and place in a small non-stick roasting tin. Spoon the remaining yogurt mixture over the chicken and wrap the vine leaves around the breast.
7 Cover with aluminium foil and bake in the oven for 20 minutes until fully cooked.

Herby Lemon Roast Chicken

SERVES 4
PER SERVING
240 CALORIES
7G FAT
PREP TIME 30 MINUTES
COOK TIME 1–1½ HOURS

1 × 1kg medium free range or
    organic chicken
2 lemons
2 tsps dried oregano
salt and freshly ground black
    pepper

1 Preheat the oven to 180C, 350F, Gas Mark 4.

Tip

Check the chicken is fully cooked by inserting a skewer into the thickest part of the joints. The juices should run out clear when fully cooked

2 Prepare the chicken by washing well inside and out. Cut away as much skin as possible from the underneath. Place the prepared chicken on a non-stick roasting tray.
3 Cut the lemons in half and squeeze the juice all over the chicken. Season with salt and black pepper and sprinkle with oregano.
4 Bake the chicken in the middle of the oven for 1–1½ hours until fully cooked, or follow the time specified on the packaging.
5 When cooked, remove from the oven and cover with foil. Allow to stand for 10 minutes before carving.

Mango and Mushroom Chicken Stir-Fry

SERVES 4
PER SERVING
228 CALORIES
3.5G FAT
PREP TIME 10 MINUTES
MARINATING TIME 1 HOUR
COOK TIME 20 MINUTES

450g skinned and boned chicken breast
225g chestnut mushrooms, sliced
1 tbsp chopped fresh coriander
salt and freshly ground black pepper

for the marinade
zest and juice of 1 lime
2 tbsps soy sauce
2 garlic cloves, crushed
2 tbsps mango chutney
150ml/¼ pint tomato passata

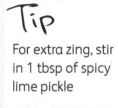

Tip

For extra zing, stir in 1 tbsp of spicy lime pickle

1 Cut the chicken into small cubes and place in a shallow dish.
2 Combine the marinade ingredients and pour over the chicken. Allow to marinate for 1 hour.
3 Heat a non-stick wok. Add the chicken and dry-fry quickly over a high heat for 5–6 minutes, turning frequently. Add the mushrooms and continue cooking for 10 minutes. Just before serving stir in the fresh coriander.

Marinated Barbecue Chicken ❁

SERVES 4
PER SERVING
293 CALORIES
12G FAT
PREP TIME 20 MINUTES
MARINATING TIME 1 HOUR
COOK TIME 30 MINUTES

8 × 225g chicken joints (legs and thighs)

for the marinade
2 tbsps tomato purée
2 tsps soft dark brown sugar
2 tbsps balsamic vinegar
pinch of fennel seeds
salt and freshly ground black pepper

1 Place the chicken joints on a chopping board. Pull off the skin, using kitchen paper and a small sharp knife, and discard. Place the chicken in a mixing bowl.

2 Mix together the marinade
  ingredients in a small bowl and pour
  over the chicken. Mix well, rubbing the
  marinade into the chicken pieces.
  Season with salt and black pepper.
  Cover and leave to marinate in the
  refrigerator for an hour.
3 Cook the chicken under a hot grill for
  30 minutes, turning regularly.
  Serve hot or cold.

Tip

These barbecued
chicken joints
make great party
food

Creamy Pineapple Chicken ❄

SERVES 4
PER SERVING
268 CALORIES
10G FAT
PREP TIME 10 MINUTES
COOK TIME 30 MINUTES

4 × 150g skinned and boned chicken breasts
1 × 432g can pineapple in juice, drained
1 × 400ml can reduced-fat coconut milk
1 small red chilli
2 tsps finely chopped lemongrass
150ml/¼ pint tomato passata
1 red onion, finely sliced
2 garlic cloves, crushed
1 × 160g pack mangetout
2 tbsps chopped fresh coriander
salt and freshly ground black pepper

Tip

You can freeze
fresh lemongrass
and, when ready
to use, remove
from the freezer
and chop straight
away

1 Cut the chicken into bite-sized pieces and season with salt and black pepper.
2 Place the pineapple, coconut milk, chilli, lemongrass and passata into a liquidiser and blend until smooth.
3 Heat a large, non-stick pan, add the onion and garlic and dry-fry until soft. Add the chicken and continue cooking until the chicken has changed colour.
4 Pour the sauce into the pan and simmer gently for 15 minutes until the chicken is cooked through.
5 Just before serving stir in the mangetout and coriander.

Turkey and Pepper Burgers ❉

SERVES 4
PER SERVING
142 CALORIES
2.2G FAT
PREP TIME 15 MINUTES
COOK TIME 25 MINUTES

450g extra lean minced turkey
1 medium red onion, finely chopped
1 garlic clove, crushed
½ red pepper, finely chopped
2 tsps vegetable stock powder
6 basil leaves, finely chopped
freshly ground black pepper

Tip
Make the burgers in advance and store in the refrigerator for up to 3 days

1 In a large mixing bowl combine the turkey mince, onion, garlic and red pepper, working the mixture with 2 forks to break up the meat.

2 Sprinkle the stock powder over and stir in well, making sure the mixture is fully combined.

3 Add the chopped basil leaves and season with plenty of freshly ground black pepper. Mix well, using your hands, and bring the mixture together. Form into burger shapes, squeezing the mixture between your hands to form a tight ball and then flatten slightly. Set aside.

4 Cook the burgers under a hot grill for 10 minutes each side. Make sure the burgers are cooked. Pull one apart to check the centre is fully cooked. If in doubt, return to the grill.

Spicy Chicken Pasta

SERVES 4
PER SERVING
398 CALORIES
3.3G FAT
PREP TIME 10 MINUTES
COOK TIME 20 MINUTES

225g (uncooked weight) tagliatelle
1 vegetable stock cube
1 red onion, finely chopped
2 garlic cloves, crushed
1 red pepper, seeded and finely sliced
4 × 100g skinless chicken breasts, cut into strips
1 × 400g can chopped tomatoes
1 red chilli, seeded and finely chopped
8–10 basil leaves, shredded
salt and freshly ground black pepper
Parmesan cheese, to serve

Tip

To cool down this spicy sauce slightly, stir in a little virtually fat free fromage frais just before serving. This also results in a creamier sauce

1 Cook the pasta in boiling water with a vegetable stock cube.
2 In a non-stick frying pan dry-fry the onion for 2–3 minutes until soft. Add the garlic and red pepper and cook for a further 2–3 minutes.
3 Add the chicken strips and season with salt and black pepper. Cook for 5 minutes until the chicken is firm and changes colour. Turn during cooking so that the chicken strips cook on all sides.
4 Add the tomatoes and chilli and bring to a gentle simmer.
5 Drain the pasta and pour into a serving dish. Spoon the sauce over and sprinkle with shredded basil leaves and a little Parmesan.

Turkey and Bacon Hotpot ❋

SERVES 4
PER SERVING
412 CALORIES
6.4G FAT
PREP TIME 20 MINUTES
COOK TIME 20–30 MINUTES

2 red onions
2 garlic cloves, crushed
450g lean diced turkey
225g thick-cut lean bacon, diced
1 tbsp sauce flour or plain flour
450ml semi-skimmed milk
1 chicken stock cube
1 tbsp chopped fresh parsley
450g potatoes, peeled and thinly sliced
1 tbsp reduced-salt soy sauce
freshly ground black pepper

1 Preheat the oven to 190C, 375F, Gas Mark 5.
2 Heat a non-stick frying pan. Add the onions and garlic and dry-fry until soft.
3 Add the turkey and bacon and continue cooking, turning the meat to seal on all sides.
4 Sprinkle the flour over and 'cook out' for 1 minute, then gradually stir in the milk and the stock cube. Simmer gently for 15 minutes to allow the sauce to thicken.
5 Stir in the parsley and spoon the mixture into an ovenproof dish. Top with the sliced potatoes, drizzle with the soy sauce and season with freshly ground black pepper.
6 Bake in the oven for 20–30 minutes until the potatoes are cooked.

Tip

To speed up the oven cooking time, parboil the potatoes in boiling water for 5 minutes, drain and allow to cool before slicing

Pan-Fried Duck with Black Bean Sauce

SERVES 4
PER SERVING
155 CALORIES
6G FAT
PREP TIME 10 MINUTES
MARINATING TIME 1 HOUR
COOK TIME 20 MINUTES

2 × 150g duck breasts
150ml pineapple juice
2 tbsps chopped fresh coriander

for the marinade
2 garlic cloves, crushed
1 tbsp sweet chilli sauce
2 tbsps light soy sauce
1 × 2.5cm piece fresh ginger, peeled and finely chopped
2 tbsps black bean sauce

1　Using a sharp knife, remove the skin from the duck.
2　Place the marinade ingredients in a large bowl and mix well. Add the duck and mix well to coat with the marinade. Leave to marinate for at least 1 hour.
3　Heat a non-stick griddle pan. Remove the duck from the marinade (reserve the marinade), add to the pan and cook for 4–5 minutes on each side, depending on the thickness of the breasts. Remove from pan, place on a chopping board and allow to rest for 5 minutes.
4　Pour the reserved marinade into the pan and add the pineapple juice. Simmer gently for 5 minutes until the sauce thickens.
5　Slice the duck and sprinkle with chopped coriander.

Tip

For maximum flavour, marinate the duck overnight

Beef

Crispy Steak and Kidney Pie ✱

SERVES 4
PER SERVING
262 CALORIES
7.4G FAT
PREP TIME 10 MINUTES
COOK TIME 1 HOUR

450g lean steak and kidney
1 red onion, finely chopped
1 tbsp chopped fresh thyme
1–2 tbsps gravy granules
6 sheets filo pastry
1 egg, beaten with 1 tbsp semi-skimmed milk

> **Tip**
> Cover the filo pastry with damp kitchen towel to prevent it drying out while you assemble the pie

1 Chop the steak and kidney into pieces and place in a saucepan with the onion and thyme. Just cover with water and bring to a gentle simmer.
2 Stir in the gravy granules until the gravy starts to thicken. Reduce the heat and simmer until the meat is tender. Allow to cool slightly.
3 Preheat the oven to 200C, 400F, Gas Mark 6.
4 Once the meat has cooled a little, use a slotted spoon to spoon it into the bottom of an ovenproof dish.
5 Take a sheet of filo pastry, brush lightly with the milk and egg mixture and carefully place over the meat. Repeat with the other sheets, and then trim the pastry around the outside of the dish with scissors.
6 Bake in the oven for 15–20 minutes until golden brown.

Fillet Steak with Redcurrant and Thyme Glaze

SERVES 1
PER SERVING
215 CALORIES
6G FAT
PREP TIME 10 MINUTES
COOK TIME 20 MINUTES

1 × 150g lean rump steak
2 tsps redcurrant jelly
½ tsp chopped fresh thyme
40ml vegetable stock
salt and freshly ground black pepper

1 Heat a non-stick frying pan. Season the steak on both sides with salt and black pepper. Add to the pan and seal for 2–3 minutes on each side. Continue cooking for a further 5 minutes, turning the steak regularly. Remove from the pan and keep warm.
2 Add the redcurrant jelly, thyme and stock to the pan and mix well. Simmer gently to allow the sauce to thicken then return the steak to the pan to coat with the glaze before serving.

Tip

Use a health grill or griddle pan sprayed with a little low-calorie cooking sprayl to sear the steak if you like to see grill marks

Grilled Steak Verde

SERVES 4
PER SERVING
319 CALORIES
10G FAT
PREP TIME 5 MINUTES
COOK TIME 6–10 MINUTES

4 × 175g lean beef steaks
1 green pepper, seeded and diced
1 garlic clove, crushed
1 tbsp chopped fresh mint
1 tbsp chopped fresh parsley
50g gherkins, chopped
salt and freshly ground black pepper

1 Preheat the grill to high.
2 Season the steaks on both sides with salt and black pepper
   and place under the hot grill to cook for 3–5 minutes on
   each side.
3 Meanwhile, place the remaining ingredients in a bowl, mix
   well and season with salt and black pepper.
4 Just before the steaks are fully cooked, remove from the
   grill and spoon the sauce on top.
5 Return to the grill and heat through
   for 1–2 minutes.

Tip

Try this versatile
green sauce with
cold meats and
pasta

Creamy Madeira Beef ❄

SERVES 4
PER SERVING
307 CALORIES
10G FAT
PREP TIME 10 MINUTES
COOK TIME 40–45 MINUTES

4 × 150g lean braising steaks
1 medium red onion, finely chopped
1 × 2.5cm piece fresh ginger, peeled
    and finely chopped
1 beef stock cube, dissolved in
    300ml/½ pint boiling water
1 tbsp plain flour
225g chestnut mushrooms, sliced
1 wine glass Madeira wine
2 tbsps chopped fresh mixed herbs

Tip

Before cooking, beat the steaks lightly with a rolling pin. This will help to tenderise the meat, which reduces the cooking time

1 Heat a non-stick frying pan. Season the steaks on both sides with salt and black pepper then place in the pan. Dry-fry on each side for 5–6 minutes until lightly browned. Remove from the pan and place on a plate.
2 Add the onion to the pan and cook gently until lightly coloured. Add the ginger and 2 tbsps of stock. Sprinkle the flour over and 'cook out' for 1 minute. Gradually stir in the remaining stock. Add the mushrooms and wine.
3 Return the beef to the pan and add the herbs. Simmer gently for 35–40 minutes until the sauce has reduced and the beef is tender.

Boozy Beef with Mushrooms ❄

SERVES 4
PER SERVING
230 CALORIES
7.1G FAT
PREP TIME 10 MINUTES
COOK TIME 50 MINUTES

2 red onions, sliced
2 garlic cloves, crushed
450g lean braising steak, diced
1 beef stock cube, dissolved in 300ml/½ pint boiling water
1 tbsp plain flour
225g mixed mushrooms, sliced
300ml/½ pint beer or cider
2 tbsps chopped fresh mixed herbs
salt and freshly ground black pepper

1 Heat a large, non-stick pan, add the sliced red onions and
   dry-fry until brown. Add the garlic and beef steak, and
   continue cooking to seal the beef, seasoning with salt and
   black pepper.
2 Add 2 tbsps of beef stock and sprinkle
   the flour over. Mix well and 'cook out'
   for 1 minute before gradually stirring in
   the remaining stock.
3 Stir in the sliced mushrooms, the beer
   or cider and the herbs.
4 Reduce the heat to a gentle simmer
   and cook for 35–40 minutes until the
   beef is tender.

Tip

For added
flavour, marinate
the meat in the
beer overnight
before cooking

Beef and Root Vegetable Stew ❄

SERVES 4
PER SERVING
289 CALORIES
7.7G FAT
PREP TIME 10 MINUTES
COOK TIME 1 HOUR 20 MINUTES

2 red onions, diced
2 garlic cloves, crushed
450g lean diced beef
1 tbsp flour
1.2 litres/2 pints beef stock
450g small new potatoes
2 celery sticks, chopped
1 swede, peeled and diced
1 tbsp chopped fresh herbs (parsley, thyme, chives)
salt and freshly ground black pepper

1 Heat a non-stick frying pan, add the onions and garlic and
   dry-fry until the onion starts to brown.
2 Add the beef and season with salt and black pepper.
   Continue cooking to seal the beef.
3 Sprinkle the flour over and 'cook out'
   for 1 minute.
4 Gradually stir in the meat stock.
5 Add the vegetables and herbs, cover
   and simmer gently for 1 hour until the
   meat is tender.

Tip

Choose lean braising steak and remove all visible fat before cooking

Braised Beef with Tomatoes and Thyme ❄

SERVES 4
PER SERVING
265 CALORIES
5.9G FAT
PREP TIME 10 MINUTES
COOK TIME 1 HOUR

4 × 125g extra lean beef steaks
2 medium onions, finely chopped
2 garlic cloves, crushed
2 tsps chopped fresh thyme
150ml/¼ pint strong beef stock
2 × 400g cans chopped tomatoes
225g baby carrots, sliced lengthways
225g mushrooms, cut into quarters
salt and freshly ground black pepper
2 tbsps chopped fresh parsley,
    to garnish

1 Preheat the oven to 180C, 350F, Gas Mark 4.
2 Season both sides of the steaks with salt and black pepper and place in a preheated non-stick frying pan. Seal on each side until lightly browned, then transfer to an ovenproof dish.
3 Wipe out any excess fat from the pan, using absorbent kitchen paper, then add the onions, garlic and thyme cook gently for 2–3 minutes until soft.

Tip

If the steaks are thick, place on a chopping board and bash with a rolling pin. This will tenderise them and speed up the cooking time

4 Stir in the stock, then add the tomatoes and vegetables. Pour the sauce over the steaks, cover and place in the oven for 35–40 minutes until the sauce has reduced and the meat is tender.

5 Garnish with fresh parsley before serving.

Thai Beef Stir-Fry ✳

SERVES 4
PER SERVING
179 CALORIES
5.5G FAT
PREP TIME 10 MINUTES
COOK TIME 10 MINUTES

450g lean rump or sirloin steak
2 tsps ground coriander
1 red onion, finely chopped
2 garlic cloves, crushed
1 × 5cm piece lemongrass, finely chopped
1 small red chilli, sliced
4 Kaffir lime leaves
300ml tomato passata
1 beef stock cube
1 tbsp chopped fresh coriander
1 tbsp horseradish sauce
salt and freshly ground black pepper

> **Tip**
> You can substitute strips of chicken, turkey or lean pork for the beef

1 Remove any visible fat from the meat. Slice the meat into thin strips and place in a shallow dish. Season with salt and black pepper and coat with the ground coriander.

2 Heat a non-stick wok. Add the onion and garlic and dry-fry until soft. Add the coated meat and cook quickly over a high heat.

3 Add the lemongrass, sliced chilli and lime leaves and toss the ingredients together. Stir in the tomato passata, crumble the stock cube into the pan, and heat through.

4 Remove the pan from the heat and stir in the fresh coriander and horseradish sauce.

Easy Beef Curry ❈

SERVES 4
PER SERVING
263 CALORIES
9G FAT
PREP TIME 10 MINUTES
COOK TIME 30 MINUTES

2 red onions, sliced
2 garlic cloves, crushed
450g lean beef steak, diced
2 tbsps medium curry powder
2 × 400g cans chopped tomatoes
4 Kaffir lime leaves or curry leaves
1 tbsp lime pickle
1 tbsp mango chutney
2 tsps vegetable stock powder
salt and freshly ground black pepper
2 tbsps chopped fresh coriander, to garnish

> **Tip**
>
> Browning the onions adds more flavour to the finished dish

1 Heat a large non-stick pan. Add the red onions and dry-fry until brown.

2 Add the garlic and the beef steak, and continue cooking to seal the beef. Mix in the curry powder and cook for a further minute.

3 Stir in the tomatoes and then add the remaining ingredients except the coriander. Reduce the heat and simmer gently for 20 minutes until the beef is tender.

4 Garnish with the coriander before serving.

Beef Masala ✳

SERVES 4
PER SERVING
207 CALORIES
4.9G FAT
PREP TIME 15 MINUTES
COOK TIME 1 HOUR

450g lean stewing steak
1 red onion, finely chopped
2 garlic cloves, crushed
few drops light soy sauce
1 tbsp chopped fresh thyme
1 tbsp madras curry powder
2 × 400g cans chopped tomatoes
1 beef stock cube
6 cardamom pods, seeds removed
2–3 tbsps low-fat natural yogurt
salt and freshly ground black pepper
chopped fresh coriander, to garnish

1 Preheat a non-stick frying pan.
2 Chop the steak into cubes.

Tip

Adding a little soy sauce when dry-frying beef enhances the flavour and prevents the meat from drying out

3 Add the onion and garlic to the hot pan and dry-fry until the onion starts to colour.
4 Add the beef and soy sauce to the pan. Stir in the thyme and curry powder. Add the tomatoes, stock cube and cardamom seeds and stir well. Allow to simmer gently until the meat is tender and the sauce has reduced.
5 Spoon into a serving dish, drizzle with the yogurt and sprinkle with the coriander.

Beef Stroganoff

SERVES 4
PER SERVING
215 CALORIES
5.6G FAT
PREP TIME 10 MINUTES
COOK TIME 30 MINUTES

450g lean rump steak
1 red onion, finely chopped
2 garlic cloves, crushed
1 tbsp chopped fresh thyme
300ml/½ pint beef stock
1 tbsp plain flour
225g mushrooms, sliced
2 tsps Dijon mustard
300ml/½ pint virtually fat free fromage frais
2 tbsps chopped fresh parsley
2 tbsps brandy
salt and freshly ground black pepper

1 Preheat a non-stick frying pan.
2 Chop the steak into cubes. Add the onion and garlic to the hot pan and dry-fry until soft.
3 Add the beef and thyme and cook to seal the outside of the meat. Add a little stock and sprinkle the flour over. Mix well, and 'cook out' the flour for 1 minute before adding the remaining stock.
4 Add the mushrooms, stir in the mustard and cook for a further 3–4 minutes.
5 Remove the pan from the heat and stir in the fromage frais and parsley. Check the seasoning and adjust if necessary.
6 Heat the brandy in a ladle held over a low heat and carefully light the top of the alcohol. Pour the flaming brandy into the pan and stir in. Serve immediately.

Tip

Flaming the alcohol takes away the bitter edge from the sauce and gives a more mellow flavour

Beef and Mushroom Skewers

SERVES 4
PER SERVING
148 CALORIES
4.8G FAT
PREP TIME 10 MINUTES
COOK TIME 5–8 MINUTES

350g extra thin lean beef steaks
1 red pepper, seeded
16 chestnut mushrooms

for the sauce
2 tbsps horseradish sauce
2 tbsps light soy sauce
1 tbsp chopped fresh parsley

1 Cut the steaks into thin strips and the red pepper into chunks. Thread the beef strips, concertina-style, onto 8 large skewers, placing a chunk of red pepper and a mushroom between each strip.
2 Mix together the sauce ingredients in a small bowl, and add a little boiling water to form a coating consistency.
3 Preheat the grill to high. Place the skewers on a grill tray and brush lightly with the sauce.
4 Cook under the hot grill for 5–8 minutes, basting occasionally with the sauce. Serve straight from the grill.

Tip

For an extra peppery flavour, sprinkle the beef with crushed mixed peppercorns before cooking

Paprika Mince ❄

SERVES 4
PER SERVING
300 CALORIES
10G FAT
PREP TIME 10 MINUTES
COOK TIME 35 MINUTES

675g extra lean minced beef
2 carrots, chopped
2 celery sticks, chopped
2 red onions, finely diced
1 tbsp chopped fresh oregano
1 tbsp paprika
600ml/1 pint beef stock
1 tbsp gravy granules
salt and freshly ground black pepper

1 Heat a non-stick frying pan. Add the mince and dry-fry until
   cooked through. Drain off any excess fat.
2 Add the carrots, celery sticks and onions to the pan and stir
   in the oregano and paprika. Cook for 2–3 minutes.
3 Add the beef stock and simmer gently, while stirring in the
   gravy granules. Cover with a lid and simmer for 20 minutes
   until the meat is tender.
4 Adjust the seasoning and serve.

Tip

Make this dish a
day in advance
and reheat as
required

Savoury Meatloaf with Caramelised Onion Gravy ❄

SERVES 6
PER SERVING
316 CALORIES
6.5G FAT
PREP TIME 10 MINUTES
COOK TIME 1 HOUR 10 MINUTES

for the meatloaf
225g lean minced beef
225g lean minced pork
50g fresh breadcrumbs
2 tbsps chopped fresh mixed herbs (parsley, thyme, oregano)
1 small red onion, finely chopped
1 eating apple, grated
salt and freshly ground black pepper

for the onion gravy
2 red onions, finely sliced
1 tsp runny honey
2–3 tsps gravy powder
1 tsp wholegrain mustard
1 tbsp finely chopped fresh chives

1 Preheat the oven to 190C, 375F, Gas Mark 5.
2 Mix all the meatloaf ingredients together in a large bowl
   and season with salt and black pepper.
3 Press the mixture into a 450g loaf tin or individual ramekin
   dishes. Stand the tin or ramekins in a roasting tin and pour
   sufficient water around to come halfway up the sides.

4 Cover with foil and bake in the oven for 1 hour.

5 To make the onion gravy, heat a non-stick pan, add the onions and runny honey and dry-fry over a moderate heat until the onions start to brown.

6 Pour 300ml/½ pint water into the pan. Mix the gravy powder with a little cold water and stir into the pan. Simmer gently and allow to thicken, adding a little more water if required, then stir in the mustard and chives.

7 Turn the meatloaf out onto a serving plate and pour some of the onion gravy over the top. Serve with the remainder of the gravy.

Tip

This recipe freezes well. Defrost overnight in the refrigerator

Lamb

Lamb Chasseur ❄

SERVES 4
PER SERVING
328 CALORIES
11G FAT
PREP TIME 15 MINUTES
COOK TIME 40 MINUTES

1 × 450g leg of lamb, skin removed
2 medium red onions, sliced
2 garlic cloves, crushed
150ml vegetable stock
1 tbsp plain flour
150ml red wine
1 × 400g can chopped tomatoes
1 tbsp chopped fresh tarragon
115g button mushrooms
salt and freshly ground black pepper
1 tbsp chopped fresh parsley, to garnish

Tip

Allow the meat to stand for 10 minutes before carving. This helps the joint relax, making it easier to carve and less tough

1   Preheat the oven to 180C, 350F, Gas Mark 4.
2   Heat a non-stick frying pan until very hot. Add the lamb and quickly brown on all sides, then transfer the meat to an earthenware dish.
3   Add the onions and garlic to the frying pan and cook until lightly coloured. Add 2–3 tbsps of vegetable stock and sprinkle the flour over. Cook briefly, then gradually mix in the remaining stock, red wine and chopped tomatoes. Bring to the boil and stir in the tarragon and mushrooms.

4 Pour the sauce over the lamb and cover with a lid.

5 Place in the oven and bake for 40 minutes until tender.

6 Before serving, scoop any fat from the top of the dish with a small ladle, then remove the lamb from the sauce and place on a serving plate. Spoon the sauce into a saucepan and reduce over a high heat.

7 Serve the lamb with the sauce.

Minted Lamb Samosas

SERVES 4
PER SERVING (3 SAMOSAS)
205 CALORIES
8G FAT
PREP TIME 20 MINUTES
COOK TIME 15–20 MINUTES

225g lean minced lamb
1 medium onion, finely chopped
1 garlic clove, crushed
2 tsps vegetable stock powder
1 tbsp chopped fresh mint
1 tbsp mango chutney
4 sheets filo pastry
low-calorie cooking spray
salt and freshly ground black pepper

1 Preheat the oven to 200C, 400F, Gas Mark 6.

2 Heat a non-stick frying pan, add the lamb and dry-fry until lightly browned. Pour into a sieve and remove any fat. Wipe out the pan with kitchen paper and add the onion and garlic. Dry-fry for 2–3 minutes until soft.

3 Return the lamb to the pan, add the stock powder, mint and chutney and mix well. Remove from the heat and allow to cool.
4 Place the filo sheets on a chopping board. Cut each sheet into three lengthways. Lightly spray with cooking spray then place 2 tsps of the lamb mixture at each end of the 3 strips. Fold the pastry over diagonally, enclosing the meat in a triangle. Arrange on a baking tray and spray with oil.
5 Bake in the oven for 15–20 minutes until golden brown.

Tip

These tasty pastry triangles make ideal party food. Prepare in advance and just warm through in the oven

Fillet of Lamb with Minted Couscous

SERVES 4
PER SERVING
367 CALORIES
16.6G FAT
PREP TIME 10 MINUTES
COOK TIME 20 MINUTES

450g lamb fillet
2 tbsps redcurrant jelly
400ml vegetable stock
2 tsps ground coriander
2 tsps ground cumin
175g couscous
1 tbsp chopped fresh mint
4 tomatoes, skinned, seeded and chopped
salt and freshly ground black pepper

1 Preheat the grill to hot.
2 Place the lamb on a baking tray and season with salt and black pepper.
3 Heat the redcurrant jelly in a small saucepan or microwave. Pour over the lamb and baste the lamb all over, using a pastry brush.
4 Cook under the hot grill for 10–15 minutes according to the thickness of the fillet. Remove from the grill, cover with foil and allow to rest for 5 minutes.
5 Meanwhile, bring the vegetable stock to the boil and add the spices. Add the couscous, remove from the heat and cover with a lid. Leave to steam for 1 minute then fluff up the grains with a fork. Stir in the chopped mint and tomatoes and pile onto a serving plate.
6 Carve the lamb into thin slices and arrange on top of the couscous.

 Make up the couscous in advance and reheat either in a steamer or in the microwave

Tunisian Lamb

SERVES 4
PER SERVING
255 CALORIES
9G FAT
PREP TIME 10 MINUTES
COOK TIME 40 MINUTES

1 large red onion, finely sliced
450g lean diced lamb
2 garlic cloves, chopped
1 tsp coriander seeds
1 tsp ground cumin
1 tsp ground cinnamon
½ tsp cayenne pepper
6 cardamom pods, crushed with seeds removed
300ml/½ pint meat or vegetable stock
2 tbsps plain flour
1 tbsp chopped fresh oregano
1 × 400g can chopped tomatoes
2 pieces orange peel
150ml/¼ pint orange juice
salt and freshly ground black pepper

1 Heat a non-stick frying pan. Add the
   onion and dry-fry for 2–3 minutes until
   soft. Add the lamb and garlic and cook
   briskly, turning the meat regularly to
   seal on all sides.

2 Add the spices with 2–3 tbsps of stock and sprinkle the
   flour over. Mix well and 'cook out' the flour for 1 minute.

Tip

For a vegetarian
option, substitute
Quorn pieces or
soya chunks for
the lamb

3 Gradually mix in the remaining stock. Add the oregano, tomatoes, orange peel and juice. Cover and simmer gently for 40 minutes.
4 Season to taste and serve hot.

Spicy Lamb with Sweet Potatoes ✱

Serves 4
PER SERVING
334 CALORIES
9.5G FAT
PREP TIME 15 MINUTES
COOK TIME 2 HOURS 15 MINUTES

2 red onions, chopped
2 garlic cloves, crushed
450g lean diced lamb
1 tbsp medium curry powder
1 tbsp flour
450ml vegetable stock
450g sweet potatoes, peeled and chopped
1 × 400g can chopped tomatoes
salt and freshly ground black pepper

1 Preheat the oven to 180C, 350F, Gas Mark 4.
2 Heat a non-stick frying pan. Add the onions and garlic and dry-fry until soft.
3 Add the lamb and continue cooking, turning the meat to seal on all sides. Sprinkle the curry powder and flour over and 'cook out' for 1 minute.

4 Gradually stir in the vegetable stock. Add the sweet potatoes and tomatoes and bring the sauce to a simmer. Season with salt and black pepper and transfer to a casserole dish.

5 Cover, and cook in the oven for 1½–2 hours until the meat is tender. Serve from the pot.

Tip

For a milder curry stir in a little low-fat yogurt before serving

Pork and gammon

Stir-Fried Pork with Peppers

SERVES 4
PER SERVING
266 CALORIES
4.9G FAT
PREP TIME 5 MINUTES
MARINATING TIME 20 MINUTES
COOK TIME 20 MINUTES

450g lean pork tenderloin, thinly sliced
1 red pepper, seeded and sliced
1 yellow pepper, seeded and sliced
12 spring onions, sliced

for the marinade
4 tbsps dark soy sauce
2 tbsps clear honey
2 garlic cloves, crushed
1 small red chilli, sliced

Tip

For a fuller flavour, allow the pork to marinate overnight in the refrigerator

1 In a large bowl mix together the marinade ingredients. Add the pork and stir to ensure the meat is evenly coated. Cover, and leave to marinate in the refrigerator for 20 minutes.
2 Heat a non-stick wok or large non-stick frying pan. Drain the pork, reserving the marinade, and add to the pan. Stir-fry the pork until the meat starts to firm up.
3 Add the peppers and spring onions, along with the reserved marinade. Mix well and heat through.

Pork and Pineapple Kebabs

SERVES 1
PER SERVING
309 CALORIES
6G FAT
PREP TIME 20 MINUTES
COOK TIME 20–25 MINUTES

1 × 150g lean pork steak
1 small pack chopped fresh pineapple
1 small garlic clove, finely chopped
½ small red chilli, sliced
2 tsps maple syrup
salt and freshly ground black pepper

1 Trim any visible fat off the pork steak and discard. Cut the
   steak into bite-sized pieces.
2 Take 2 skewers and thread alternate pieces of pork and
   pineapple onto each. Place in a shallow dish.
3 Mix together the garlic, chilli and
   maple syrup and pour over the
   kebabs. Season with salt and black
   pepper.
5 Place under a hot grill for 20–25
   minutes until fully cooked.
6 Serve any remaining sweet chilli
   sauce separately.

Tip

You can also cook
these kebabs on
a hot barbecue.
Use wooden
skewers soaked in
water to prevent
them from
scorching

Lime and Ginger Stir-Fried Pork

SERVES 4
PER SERVING
254 CALORIES
4.8G FAT
PREP TIME 10 MINUTES
MARINATING TIME 1 HOUR
COOK TIME 2–3 MINUTES

450g lean pork tenderloin
225g pak choi or dark cabbage
salt and freshly ground black pepper
wedges of lime, to garnish

for the marinade
2 tbsps dry sherry
zest and juice of 1 lime
1 × 2.5cm piece fresh ginger,
   peeled and finely grated
2 tbsps runny honey
2 tbsps plum sauce
1 small red chilli, sliced
2 garlic cloves, crushed
1 tbsp tomato purée

> **Tip**
>
> For a fuller flavour, leave the pork to marinate overnight in the refrigerator

1 Cut the pork into thin strips and place in a shallow dish.
2 Mix together the marinade ingredients combining them well. Pour over the pork, cover, and refrigerate. Leave to marinate for 1 hour.
3 Heat a large, non-stick frying pan, add the pak choi and cook over a high heat for 2–3 minutes. Season with salt and black pepper. Spoon into a serving dish and keep warm.

4 Return the pan to the heat. Remove the pork from the
   marinade (reserve the marinade), add to the pan and cook
   quickly over a high heat. Add the marinade and heat
   through. Spoon onto the pak choi. Garnish with the lime
   wedges.

Passionate Pork Casserole ❅

SERVES 4
PER SERVING
218 CALORIES
5.1G FAT
PREP TIME 10 MINUTES
COOK TIME 50 MINUTES

Tip

This casserole is
ideal for cooking
in a slow cooker

1 red onion, chopped
2 garlic cloves, crushed
450g lean diced pork
1 × 2cm piece fresh ginger, peeled and finely chopped
1–2 tsps vegetable stock powder
300ml/½ pint tomato passata
300ml/½ pint passion fruit or mango juice
1 tbsp runny honey
salt and freshly ground black pepper

1 Heat a large, non-stick frying pan or wok. Add the onion
   and garlic and dry-fry until soft.
2 Add the diced pork and continue cooking to seal the meat.
   Add the remaining ingredients and mix well, adding a little
   water, depending on the thickness of the passata.
3 Cover with a lid and simmer gently for a minimum of 40
   minutes until the meat is tender.

Sweet and Sour Pork Slices

SERVES 4
PER SERVING
176 CALORIES
5G FAT
PREP TIME 5 MINUTES
MARINATING TIME 30 MINUTES
COOK TIME 12–16 MINUTES

4 × 125g lean pork slices
1 small red onion, finely chopped
3 tbsps tomato passata
1 tbsp balsamic vinegar
2 tsps wholegrain mustard
1 tbsp runny honey
salt and freshly ground black pepper

1 Place the pork slices in the bottom of a shallow dish and
   season with salt and pepper.
2 In a separate bowl, combine the other ingredients. Spread
   over the pork slices, coating both sides, and leave to
   marinate for 30 minutes.
3 Cook the marinated pork under a hot
   grill for 6–8 minutes on each side.

Tip

Leave the pork
to marinate
overnight for
extra flavour

Leek, Pea, Smoked Ham and Cheese Pasta

SERVES 1
PER SERVING
255 CALORIES
6G FAT
PREP TIME 10 MINUTES
COOK TIME 25 MINUTES

50g (uncooked weight) pasta shapes
1 vegetable stock cube
40g frozen peas
2 baby leeks, finely chopped
1 garlic clove, crushed
1 slice smoked ham, chopped
50g Philadelphia Extra Light soft cheese
a few Parmesan shavings
salt and freshly ground black pepper

1 Cook the pasta in a pan of boiling water containing the vegetable stock cube, adding the frozen peas for the last 3 minutes of cooking. Drain and pour boiling water from the kettle over the pasta to rinse away the starch. Return the pasta to the pan.
2 Heat a non-stick wok or large frying pan, add the leeks and garlic and dry-fry for 1–2 minutes. Add the smoked ham and soft cheese and cook for a further minute.

Tip

Vegetarians can omit the ham and substitute 30g vegetarian cheese

3 Add the cooked pasta and toss all the ingredients together. Season with black pepper and a little salt if required.
4 Once the pasta is heated through, transfer to a warmed serving dish, sprinkle with a few Parmesan shavings and serve immediately.

Simple Citrus Gammon

SERVES 4
PER SERVING
207 CALORIES
9G FAT
PREP TIME 5 MINUTES
COOK TIME 20 MINUTES

4 × 125g gammon steaks
salt and freshly ground black pepper

for the sauce
1 × 400 can chopped tomatoes
zest and juice of 1 lemon
1 tsp vegetable stock powder
1 tbsp mixed fresh herbs

Tip

Gammon is a great standby for a quick meal – store frozen and defrost in a bowl of water

1 Season the gammon steaks with salt and black pepper. Place under a hot grill for 15 minutes, turning them regularly during cooking.
2 Meanwhile, put the sauce ingredients in a food processor and blend until smooth. Pour into a saucepan and heat.
3 Serve the steaks with the accompanying sauce.

Gammon and Pineapple Stir-Fry

SERVES 4
PER SERVING
181 CALORIES
7.3G FAT
PREP TIME 5 MINUTES
COOK TIME 15 MINUTES

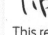

Tip

This recipe also works well with lean pork fillet or chicken

350g gammon steak
8 spring onions, finely sliced
1 red pepper, seeded and sliced
115g chestnut mushrooms, sliced
1 small can pineapple chunks in natural juice
1 tbsp cider vinegar
2 tbsp tomato purée
225g beansprouts
freshly ground black pepper

1 Remove any visible fat or rind from the gammon. Cut the gammon into thin strips.
2 Heat a non-stick wok or large, non-stick frying pan. Add the gammon strips and cook over a high heat for 2–3 minutes. Add the sliced spring onions, red pepper and mushrooms and cook for 1 minute.
4 Drain the pineapple juice into a bowl and mix with the vinegar and tomato purée.
5 Add the pineapple chunks and beansprouts to the wok and pour the sauce over them. Toss well together and bring to the boil. Serve straight from the pan.

Fish and seafood

Spiced Tomato Baked Cod ❄

SERVES 1
PER SERVING
219 CALORIES
2G FAT
PREP TIME 10 MINUTES
COOK TIME 35 MINUTES

1 × 200g cod steak, skinned
½ small red onion, finely chopped
½ garlic clove, crushed
1 large ripe tomato, diced
pinch of paprika
pinch of ground turmeric
pinch of saffron
2 tsps chopped fresh parsley
1 tsp fresh lemon juice
salt and freshly ground black pepper

Tip

For best results, choose a thick piece of cod that will retain moisture during cooking

1 Preheat the oven to 200C, 400F, Gas Mark 6.
2 Season the fish well on both sides and place, skin-side down, in an ovenproof dish.
3 Heat a non-stick frying pan, add the onion and dry-fry until soft. Add the garlic and diced tomato and cook briskly for 4–5 minutes. Add the spices and the chopped parsley and lemon juice. Season with salt and black pepper.
4 Spoon the mixture onto the cod steak and place, uncovered, in the oven for 12–15 minutes or until just cooked. The cod should flake easily when teased with a fork.

Roast Smoked Cod with Cheese and Chive Sauce

SERVES 4
PER SERVING
316 CALORIES
8.5G FAT
PREP TIME 5 MINUTES
COOK TIME 20 MINUTES

4 × 125g smoked cod steaks
1 tbsp cornflour
600ml semi-skimmed milk
1 tsp English mustard powder
1 tsp vegetable bouillon stock powder
115g low-fat mature Cheddar cheese, grated
1 tbsp chopped fresh chives

Tip

The sauce used here will keep for 3–4 days in the refrigerator. Try it with cauliflower, roast onions or drizzled on top of mash

1 Preheat the oven to 200C, 400F, Gas Mark 6.
2 Rinse the cod steaks under cold running water and place on a non-stick baking tray. Place in the oven for 12–15 minutes until cooked through. Keep warm.
3 Meanwhile, mix the cornflour with a little cold milk to a smooth paste. Pour the remaining milk into a saucepan and heat. Stir in the mustard and stock powder. Using a whisk, stir in the cornflour mix and bring the sauce to a gentle simmer. Stir in the grated cheese and chopped chives.
4 Place the cooked fish on a serving plate and spoon the sauce on top.

Smoky Prawn Stir-Fry

SERVES 4
PER SERVING
185 CALORIES
1.6G FAT
PREP TIME 10 MINUTES
COOK TIME 15 MINUTES

2 red onions, sliced
2 garlic cloves, crushed
1 red pepper, seeded and sliced
450g large peeled uncooked prawns
1 tsp smoked paprika
2 small courgettes, thinly sliced
115g chestnut mushrooms, sliced
2 tsps finely chopped fresh ginger
1 tbsp sweet chilli sauce
1 tbsp fruit chutney
juice of ½ lemon
1 tbsp runny honey
salt and freshly ground black pepper

Tip

For extra-fine sliced vegetables use a mandolin or speed peeler

1 Heat a non-stick wok. Add the onions and garlic and dry-fry until soft. Add the red pepper, prawns and paprika, toss well, and continue to cook for 2–3 minutes until the prawns are cooked through. Season with salt and black pepper.
2 Add the remaining ingredients and cook for 2 minutes, tossing them well.
3 Serve straight from the pan.

Baked Parma Ham Cod with Saffron Couscous

SERVES 4
PER SERVING
361 CALORIES
6.5G FAT
PREP TIME 5 MINUTES
COOK TIME 15–20 MINUTES

4 × 125g fresh cod fillets
8 large basil leaves
8 slices Parma ham
225g (uncooked weight) couscous
300ml/½ pint vegetable stock
pinch of saffron
1 red pepper, finely diced
salt and freshly ground black pepper
1 tbsp chopped fresh chives, to garnish

1 Preheat the oven to 200C, 400F, Gas Mark 6.
2 Place the cod fillets in an ovenproof dish. Season each fillet
   on both sides with salt and black pepper. Place 2 basil
   leaves across the top of each fillet.
   Wrap each piece of fish with 2 slices of
   Parma ham, tucking the ham neatly
   underneath the fillets.
3 Place in the oven for 15–20 minutes
   until cooked through.
4 Place the couscous in a large bowl. Add
   the saffron and red pepper.

Tip

For a tasty variation use lightly steamed asparagus in place of the cod fillets

5   Make up the stock with boiling water and pour over the couscous. Cover with a clean tea towel and allow to stand for 1 minute. Remove the tea towel and fluff up the grains with a fork.

6   Arrange the couscous on a serving plate and place the cod fillets on top. Just before serving sprinkle with the chives.

Pan-Fried Sea Bass with Wilted Spinach and Mushrooms

SERVES 4
PER SERVING
212 CALORIES
5.4G FAT
PREP TIME 15 MINUTES
COOK TIME 30 MINUTES

4 × 175g fillets of sea bass
1 red onion, finely chopped
1 garlic clove, crushed
115g chestnut mushrooms
225g fresh leaf spinach
150ml/¼ pint vegetable stock
a little soy sauce
salt and freshly ground black pepper
low-calorie cooking spray
fresh dill, to garnish

Tip

Cook the fish just before it's required as it will soon dry out and spoil if overcooked

1   Heat a shallow frying pan and lightly spray with cooking spray.

2   Season both sides of the fillets and place in the hot pan, skin-side down, and cook for 1 minute. Add the onion and

garlic and dry-fry until soft. Add the mushrooms and
continue cooking. Turn the fish over and reduce the heat.
3 Heat a non-stick wok. Add the spinach, pour a little stock
over and mix together, allowing the spinach to wilt.
4 Remove the fish from the pan and place on a serving plate
with the spinach. Drizzle a little soy sauce over the fish and
garnish with fresh dill.

Marinated Griddled Tuna

SERVES 4
PER SERVING
250 CALORIES
8G FAT
PREP TIME 10 MINUTES
MARINATING TIME 40 MINUTES
COOK TIME 4–6 MINUTES

4 × 175g thick tuna steaks

for the marinade
4 tbsps light soy sauce
zest and juice of 2 limes
1 small red chilli, seeded and finely chopped
1 × 2.5cm piece fresh ginger, peeled and finely chopped
salt and freshly ground black pepper
low-calorie cooking spray

1 Place the tuna steaks in a shallow dish and season with
black pepper.
2 Combine all the marinade ingredients in a small bowl and
pour over the tuna. Leave to marinate for 30 minutes.
3 Heat a non-stick griddle pan and lightly spray with a little
cooking spray.

4 When the pan is very hot carefully add the tuna steaks and cook quickly for 2–3 minutes on each side. Don't overcook them or the texture will become tough and dry. Serve hot.

Tip Always add fish and meat steaks to a hot pan. This seals in the flavour and retains all the juices, which prevents the food from drying out

Tuna and Tomato Pasta ✳

SERVES 4
PER SERVING
282 CALORIES
2.8G FAT
PREP TIME 10 MINUTES
COOK TIME 20 MINUTES

Tip
For a creamy pasta dish stir in 2 tbsps of virtually fat free fromage frais just before serving

225g (uncooked weight) pasta shapes
1 vegetable stock cube
8 spring onions, finely sliced
115g button mushrooms, sliced
1 × 185g can tuna in spring water, drained
300ml tomato passata
1 tbsp chopped fresh coriander
salt and freshly ground black pepper
Parmesan cheese, to serve

1 Cook the pasta in a pan of water with the stock cube.
2 Heat a non-stick frying pan. Add the spring onions and mushrooms and dry-fry for 1–2 minutes until soft.
3 Stir in the tuna and the passata and season with salt and freshly ground black pepper.

4 Drain the pasta well, return to the pan and add the tuna sauce. Sprinkle with the fresh coriander and toss well.
5 Just before serving, sprinkle with a little Parmesan cheese. Serve straight away.

Ginger Baked Smoked Salmon

SERVES 4
PER SERVING
160 CALORIES
5G FAT
PREP TIME 10 MINUTES
COOK TIME 10 MINUTES

450g smoked salmon
juice of 1 lemon
1 × 2.5cm piece fresh ginger, finely sliced
1 tsp chopped fresh dill
freshly ground black pepper
2 limes, to garnish
low-fat natural yogurt, to serve

1 Preheat the oven to 200C, 400F, Gas Mark 6.
2 Place a piece of aluminium foil over a non-stick baking tray. Place the smoked salmon down the centre of the foil and squeeze the lemon juice over the salmon. Sprinkle with the ginger and dill and season with freshly ground black pepper.
3 Fold over the foil, to enclose the salmon, and place in the oven for 10 minutes.

Tip

Use a teaspoon to peel fresh ginger. Simply scrape away the skin without wasting any of the ginger beneath

4 When cooked, remove from the oven and arrange on serving plates. Garnish each portion of salmon with half a lime. Serve with a little low-fat yogurt.

Thai Salmon Steaks

SERVES 4
PER SERVING
210 CALORIES
11G FAT
PREP TIME 10 MINUTES
COOK TIME 8–10 MINUTES

4 × 140g salmon steaks
1 garlic clove, crushed
1 tsp lemongrass paste
1 tsp ground coriander
1 small red chilli, sliced
6 basil leaves, finely chopped
2 tbsps runny honey
salt and freshly ground black pepper

1 Preheat the oven to 200C, 400F, Gas Mark 6.
2 Place the salmon steaks on a baking tray and season with salt and black pepper on both sides.
3 Mix together the remaining ingredients in a small bowl and drizzle over the steaks.
4 Bake in the oven for 8–10 minutes until just cooked.

Tip
You can serve this fragrant fish dish hot or cold

Marinated Monkfish with Fragrant Rice

SERVES 4
PER SERVING
298 CALORIES
0.8G FAT
PREP TIME 15 MINUTES
MARINATING TIME 20 MINUTES
COOK TIME 30 MINUTES

4 × 125g pieces fresh monkfish, skinned
zest and juice of 1 lime
2 tbsps low-salt soy sauce
pinch of chilli flakes
225g (uncooked weight) brown basmati rice
1 carrot, grated
30g sultanas
5 fresh basil leaves, chopped
salt and freshly ground black pepper
fresh dill, to garnish

Tip

This dish also works well with cod or haddock

1 Place the monkfish in a shallow dish. Mix together the lime, soy sauce and chilli flakes and pour over the fish. Allow to marinate for 20 minutes.
2 Meanwhile cook the basmati rice in a pan of boiling water. Drain and place in a large bowl. Add the grated carrot, sultanas and basil leaves, mix well and keep warm.
3 Place the monkfish on a baking tray and season with black pepper. Cook under the hot grill for 2–3 minutes on each side.
4 Pile the rice on a serving dish and arrange the monkfish on top. Garnish with fresh dill.

King Prawn Risotto

SERVES 4
PER SERVING
348 CALORIES
3G FAT
PREP TIME 10 MINUTES
COOK TIME 35 MINUTES

1 red onion, finely chopped
2 garlic cloves, crushed
600ml vegetable stock
1 tsp finely chopped lemongrass
225g Arborio risotto rice
450g peeled king prawns
150ml tomato passata
salt and freshly ground black pepper

1 Heat a non-stick frying pan or wok.
   Add the onion and garlic and dry-fry
   until soft.
2 In a saucepan, heat the stock and
   lemongrass to a gentle simmer.
3 When the onion is soft, add the rice.
   Gradually stir in about 450ml of the stock, allowing the rice
   to absorb it before adding more – this will take between
   15 and 20 minutes.
4 Add the prawns to the remaining stock and cook for
   2 minutes. Pour over the rice mixture. Stir in the passata.
   Adjust the consistency with a little water or extra stock, if
   necessary, and season to taste with salt and pepper.
5 Spoon into warm serving bowls and serve immediately.

Tip

For a creamy
risotto stir in 1–2
tbsps virtually fat
free fromage
frais just before
serving

Smoked Mackerel and Horseradish Pâté ❄

SERVES 4
PER SERVING
223 CALORIES
17.9G FAT
PREP TIME 10 MINUTES

225g smoked mackerel fillets
1 tbsp horseradish sauce
1 tbsp chopped fresh parsley
115g virtually fat free fromage frais
salt and freshly ground black pepper

1 Using a fork, break away the fish from the skin into a bowl.
2 Add the horseradish sauce, chopped parsley and fromage frais and mix well. Season to taste with salt and black pepper.
3 Press the mixture into a serving dish and chill until required.

Tip

Store for up to 5 days in the refrigerator or freeze until required. Also makes a great filling for jacket potatoes

Vegetarian

Parsnip and Pistachio Cutlets ⓥ

SERVES 4
PER SERVING
227 CALORIES
6.5G FAT
PREP TIME 10 MINUTES
COOK TIME 30 MINUTES

1kg parsnips, peeled
225g boiling potatoes, peeled
1 vegetable stock cube
2 onions, finely chopped
2 garlic cloves, crushed
2 tsps ground cumin
1 tsp ground coriander
2 tbsps chopped fresh mixed herbs (parsley, chives, oregano)
115g shelled pistachios
1 tsp vegetable stock powder
50g fresh breadcrumbs
salt and freshly ground black pepper

Tip

Save the stock from the cooked parsnips and potatoes and freeze to use as a base for soups and sauces

1 Boil the parsnips and potatoes together in a large saucepan of water with the stock cube. Drain well and mash until smooth.
2 Heat a heavy-based, non-stick frying pan, add the onions and garlic and dry-fry until soft. Add the spices and continue cooking for a further minute. Transfer this mixture to the saucepan containing the mash. Add the herbs, mix well and season with salt and black pepper.

3 Place the pistachios in a food processor and reduce to fine crumbs. Stir into the mash, along with the stock powder.

4 Spread the breadcrumbs out on a plate. Take a quarter of the mash mixture, form into a cutlet shape and press into the breadcrumbs. Repeat with the remaining mixture.

5 Dry-fry the cutlets in a non-stick pan or place under a preheated grill for 2–3 minutes to heat through.

Tofu Noodle Stir-Fry ⓥ

SERVES 4
PER SERVING
317 CALORIES
6.5G FAT
PREP TIME 10 MINUTES
COOK TIME 10 MINUTES

1 × 225g block tofu
2 long shallots, peeled and sliced
2 orange peppers, seeded and sliced
1 × 2.5cm piece fresh ginger, finely chopped
1 × 225g pack baby corn, carrots and mangetout
225g beansprouts
225g straight to wok noodles
1 tbsp light soy sauce
salt and freshly ground black pepper
low-calorie cooking spray
chopped fresh chives, to garnish

Tip

For added flavour add 1–2 cloves of crushed garlic to the pan while cooking the tofu

1 Drain the tofu well and pat dry with kitchen paper. Cut into pieces and season with salt and black pepper.

2 Heat a non-stick wok or pan until hot. Lightly spray with cooking spray and add the tofu. Cook quickly over a high heat, tossing the tofu pieces so that they brown evenly. Remove from the pan and place on a plate.

3 Add the shallots and peppers to the pan and cook over a high heat. Add the ginger, baby corn, carrots, mangetout and beansprouts and mix well for 2 minutes. Fold in the noodles and soy sauce until completely heated through. Return the tofu to the pan and stir well.

4 Pile into a serving dish and sprinkle with the chives.

Citrus Tofu Stir-Fry with Noodles Ⓥ

SERVES 4
PER SERVING
262 CALORIES
8.8G FAT
PREP TIME 10 MINUTES
COOK TIME 10 MINUTES

1 × 225g block tofu
115g (uncooked weight) fine noodles
2 red onions, finely sliced
2 garlic cloves, crushed
1 red pepper, seeded and finely sliced
1 × 5cm piece lemongrass, finely chopped
175g mangetout
3 tbsps orange juice
1 tbsp soy sauce
225g beansprouts
low-calorie cooking spray
salt and freshly ground black pepper

1 Cut the tofu into cubes and place on kitchen paper to drain. Heat a non-stick wok and lightly spray with cooking spray. Add the tofu and brown on all sides. Season with salt and black pepper. Transfer to a plate and set aside.
2 Cook the noodles in boiling water, then drain.
3 Return the pan to the heat, add the onions and garlic and cook for 1–2 minutes. Add the red pepper and lemongrass. Stir in the mangetout, orange juice and soy sauce and toss well together. Add the beansprouts and drained noodles, and stir well to combine. Just before serving add the tofu.

Dry the tofu well on kitchen paper, as this will help it to crisp up during cooking

Apricot and Vegetable Kebabs with Sweet Chilli Dipping Sauce Ⓥ

SERVES 4
PER SERVING
182 CALORIES
1.2G FAT
PREP TIME 20 MINUTES
COOK TIME 10 MINUTES

2 small courgettes
8 ready to eat apricots, soaked overnight
8 button mushrooms
8 cherry tomatoes
salt and freshly ground black pepper

for the sweet chilli sauce
1 tsp vegetable bouillon powder
2 tbsps dark brown sugar
1 garlic clove, crushed
1 small chilli, finely sliced
2 tbsps tomato passata
salt and freshly ground black pepper

1 Cut the courgettes into chunky wedges. Thread the
   apricots and vegetables onto skewers, place in a large
   shallow dish and season with salt and black pepper.
2 To make the sauce, dissolve the bouillon powder in 150ml/
   ¼ pint boiling water. Add the remaining sauce ingredients
   and mix until smooth. Season to taste with salt and black
   pepper.
3 Using a pastry brush, lightly brush the vegetables with the
   sauce to coat all sides.
4 Cook under a preheated hot grill for 4–5 minutes on each
   side or until lightly charred but still crisp. Brush again with
   the remaining sauce and serve immediately.

Tip
This sweet chilli
sauce also goes
well with pork

Quorn Fajitas ⓥ ❄

SERVES 4
PER SERVING
341 CALORIES
4G FAT
PREP TIME 15 MINUTES
COOK TIME 15 MINUTES

1 × 312g pack Quorn fillets
1 red onion, finely sliced
1 garlic clove, crushed
1 red pepper, seeded and sliced
1 yellow pepper, seeded and sliced
1 tsp smoked paprika
1 × 2.5cm piece fresh ginger, finely chopped
1 green chilli, thinly sliced
1 × 400g can chopped tomatoes
1 × 300g pack corn tortillas
4 tbsps low-fat natural yogurt
salt and freshly ground black pepper
1 tbsp finely chopped fresh chives,
    to garnish

Tip

The tortillas and
the prepared
Quorn mixture
can be frozen
separately

1 Preheat the oven to 180C, 350F, Gas
   Mark 4. Preheat a non-stick pan or wok.
2 Slice the Quorn fillets into bite-sized pieces.
3 Dry-fry the onion and garlic in the preheated pan until soft.
4 Add the Quorn pieces, peppers, paprika, ginger and chilli to
   the pan, and cook for a further 2–3 minutes.
5 Pour in the tomatoes, season with salt and black pepper and
   allow the sauce to simmer for about 5 minutes, until reduced.

6 Wrap the tortillas in foil and warm in the oven for 5 minutes.
7 Fill each tortilla with the Quorn mixture, drizzle a little yogurt
   on top and sprinkle with the chives. Serve immediately.

Okra and Chickpea Stew ⓥ ❄

SERVES 4
PER SERVING
194 CALORIES
5.3G FAT
PREP TIME 10 MINUTES
COOK TIME 20 MINUTES

2 red onions, chopped
2 garlic cloves, crushed
225g okra, chopped
1 red pepper, seeded and diced
1 × 400g can chopped tomatoes
2 tsps chopped fresh thyme
1–2 tsps vegetable stock powder
1 × 400g can chickpeas, drained
1 tbsp lime pickle
2 bay leaves

> ## Tip
> Okra or Ladies
> fingers are a small
> green vegetable
> best described as a
> cross between
> cucumber and
> courgette. Use
> courgettes instead
> if you wish

1 Heat a non-stick frying pan, add the onions and garlic and
   dry-fry until soft.
2 Add the chopped okra and diced red pepper and cook until
   soft.
3 Stir in the chopped tomatoes, thyme and vegetable stock
   powder. Add the drained chickpeas, lime pickle and bay
   leaves and simmer for 20 minutes.

Potato, Spinach and Cheese Bake Ⓥ ❄

SERVES 4
PER SERVING
316 CALORIES
6.5G FAT
PREP TIME 10 MINUTES
COOK TIME 25 MINUTES

1kg potatoes, peeled
2 leeks, washed and sliced
225g spinach, washed
2–3 tbsps semi-skimmed milk
115g low-fat Cheddar cheese
pinch of nutmeg
4 cherry tomatoes
salt and freshly ground black pepper

1 Preheat the oven to 200C, 400F, Gas Mark 6.
2 Boil the potatoes in a large pan of salted water until soft.
   Drain and mash, adding the leeks, spinach and milk.
3 Using a wooden spoon, fold in half the cheese along with
   the nutmeg and season to taste with salt and black pepper.
   Pile into an ovenproof dish.
4 Slice the tomatoes and arrange on top
   of the potatoes. Sprinkle with the
   remaining cheese and bake in the oven
   for 20 minutes or until golden brown.

Tip

Slice the leeks
very fine so that
they will not
need pre-cooking
before adding to
the potatoes

Beans in Red Wine Ⓥ ❄

SERVES 4
PER SERVING
362 CALORIES
2.5G FAT
PREP TIME 10 MINUTES
COOK TIME 25 MINUTES

2 red onions, finely diced
2 garlic cloves, crushed
2 celery sticks, chopped
115g red lentils
1 tbsp chopped fresh thyme
300ml/½ pint red wine
1 × 400g can chopped tomatoes
1 × 400g can kidney beans, drained and rinsed
1 × 400g can cannellini beans, drained and rinsed
1–2 tsps vegetable stock powder
salt and freshly ground black pepper

1 Heat a large, non-stick pan, add the onions and garlic and dry-fry until soft.
2 Add the chopped celery, lentils and thyme. Pour in the wine, tomatoes and beans and stir in the stock powder. Bring to the boil, then reduce the heat to a gentle simmer.
3 Simmer for 20 minutes, until the lentils are soft, adding a little water if required.
4 Season to taste with salt and black pepper and serve.

Tip

Choose a red wine with a screw top as it will be easier to store once opened

Courgette Pasta Bake ⓥ ❋

SERVES 4
PER SERVING
293 CALORIES
2G FAT
PREP TIME 15 MINUTES
COOK TIME 55 MINUTES

225g (uncooked weight) pasta shapes
1 vegetable stock cube
4 courgettes, diced
2 red onions, finely sliced
2 garlic cloves, crushed
1 red chilli, sliced
1 tbsp chopped fresh basil
600g tomato passata
3 tbsps virtually fat-free fromage frais
2 tbsps chopped fresh parsley
salt and freshly ground black pepper

Tip

Choose young, brightly coloured courgettes, as the older they are, the more bitter the flavour

1 Preheat the oven to 190C, 375F, Gas Mark 5.
2 Cook the pasta in a pan of boiling water with the stock cube, then drain.
3 Heat a large non-stick pan. Add the courgettes, onion and garlic and dry-fry for 3–4 minutes. Add the chilli, basil and tomato passata. Bring the sauce to a gentle simmer, then stir in the cooked pasta and season with salt and black pepper.
4 Transfer to an ovenproof dish and bake in the oven for 30 minutes. Just before serving, dot with the fromage frais and sprinkle with chopped fresh parsley.

Pasta with Creamy Tomato Pesto Ⓥ

SERVES 4
PER SERVING
249 CALORIES
8.9G FAT
PREP TIME 5 MINUTES
COOK TIME 20 MINUTES

50g sundried tomatoes
2 garlic cloves, crushed
1 tsp ground coriander
100g Philadelphia Extra Light soft cheese
225g (uncooked weight) tagliatelle or pappardelle pasta
1 vegetable stock cube
1 tbsp chopped fresh coriander
salt and freshly ground black pepper

1 Place the sundried tomatoes in a small saucepan. Add the garlic and cover with water. Simmer gently for 10–15 minutes until soft. Allow to cool slightly, then pour into a food processor and blend until smooth.

2 Return the tomatoes and garlic to the pan and reheat, then stir in the coriander and soft cheese.

3 Cook the pasta in a pan of water with the stock cube.

4 Drain the pasta well, return to the pan and add the sauce. Sprinkle the fresh coriander over the pasta and toss well. Serve straight away.

Tip

Pep up this pasta dish by adding a few dried chilli flakes to the pesto

Fresh Tomato and Basil Pasta ⓥ

SERVES 1
PER SERVING
366 CALORIES
1.7G FAT
PREP TIME 10 MINUTES
COOK TIME 30 MINUTES

80g (uncooked weight) pasta shapes
10 fresh basil leaves
½ garlic clove, crushed
½ tsp vegetable stock powder
1 tbsp boiling water
115g cherry tomatoes, cut in half
1 tbsp virtually fat free fromage frais
salt and freshly ground black pepper
Parmesan cheese, to serve

Tip

Add a vegetable stock cube to the pasta cooking water for extra flavour. It will also help prevent the pasta from sticking to the pan

1 Cook the pasta in boiling salted water.
2 Meanwhile, pick the basil leaves from the stems and place in a food processor. Add the garlic, stock powder and boiling water. Process until smooth.
3 Drain the pasta and pour back into the saucepan. Add the basil pesto, fromage frais and cherry tomatoes. Mix well and season with salt and black pepper.
4 Pile into a serving dish and finish with a little freshly grated Parmesan cheese.

Vegetable Pasta Stir-Fry Ⓥ

SERVES 4
PER SERVING
283 CALORIES
2.5G FAT
PREP TIME 10 MINUTES
COOK TIME 20 MINUTES

225g (uncooked weight) thin ribbon or tagliatelle pasta
1 vegetable stock cube
225g broccoli florets
2 red onions, sliced
2 garlic cloves, crushed
1 red pepper, seeded and sliced
115g sugar snap peas
115g chestnut mushrooms, sliced
salt and freshly ground black pepper

for the sauce
1 tbsp sweet chilli sauce
1 tbsp soy sauce
juice of ½ lemon
1 tbsp tomato purée

Tip

This recipe is a good way of using up packet ends of different pastas

1 Cook the pasta in a pan of boiling water with the vegetable stock cube. Just before the pasta is cooked, add the broccoli to blanch it, then drain the pasta and broccoli together in a colander and rinse with boiling water from a kettle.

2 Heat a non-stick wok. Add the onions and garlic and dry-fry until soft. Stir in the remaining vegetables and toss well. Season with salt and black pepper.

3 Add the cooked pasta and broccoli to the wok. Mix together the sauce ingredients and stir into the pan. Using 2 spoons, mix together thoroughly before serving.

Creamy Vegetable Tagliatelle Ⓥ

SERVES 4
PER SERVING
302 CALORIES
4G FAT
PREP TIME 5 MINUTES
COOK TIME 25 MINUTES

350g (uncooked weight) tagliatelle
1 vegetable stock cube
1 red onion, finely chopped
1 garlic clove, crushed
1 red pepper, seeded and diced
1 courgette, grated
75g Philadelphia Extra Light soft cheese
salt and freshly ground black pepper
2 tsps grated Parmesan cheese, to serve
fresh chives, to garnish

1 Cook the pasta in a large pan of boiling water with the stock cube.
2 Heat a non-stick frying pan, add the onion and garlic and dry-fry until soft. Add the red pepper and grated courgette and season with salt and black pepper.

Tip

When draining the pasta, pour boiling water from the kettle over it to loosen the starch

3 Stir the soft cheese into the sauce and reduce the heat.
4 Drain the pasta and place in serving bowls. Spoon the sauce on top, sprinkle with a little Parmesan and garnish with the chives.

Pasta Arrabiata ⓥ❋

SERVES 2
PER SERVING
398 CALORIES
3G FAT
PREP TIME 10 MINUTES
COOK TIME 20 MINUTES

175g (uncooked weight) penne pasta
1 vegetable stock cube
1 red onion, finely chopped
1 garlic clove, crushed
pinch of chopped fresh thyme
1 long red pepper, seeded and finely sliced
1 small red chilli, seeded and finely sliced
1 × 400g can chopped tomatoes
salt and freshly ground black pepper

Tip

The best way to store chillies is frozen – take straight from the freezer and chop as required. Freezing also removes some of the heat from the chilli

1 Cook the pasta in a pan of boiling water with the vegetable stock cube.
2 Heat a non-stick frying pan, add the onion and garlic and dry-fry until soft. Add the thyme, red pepper, chilli and chopped tomatoes. Simmer gently for 5 minutes to allow the sauce to thicken.
3 Drain the pasta and arrange in serving bowls. Pour the sauce over and serve immediately.

Vegetable Quinoa Salad ⓥ

SERVES 4
PER SERVING
108 CALORIES
2G FAT
PREP TIME 10 MINUTES
COOK TIME 15 MINUTES

100g quinoa
1 vegetable stock cube
6 spring onions, chopped
1 red pepper, diced
2 tomatoes, diced
1 courgette, finely diced
a few fresh basil leaves, finely chopped
lemon juice
salt and freshly ground black pepper

1 Place the quinoa in a small saucepan, add the vegetable stock cube and 500ml of boiling water. Bring to the boil, reduce the heat and simmer gently for 10–15 minutes until the water has been absorbed.
2 Remove from the heat and spoon the quinoa into a mixing bowl. Add the diced vegetables and chopped basil leaves and mix well. Season with salt and black pepper and a little lemon juice.
3 Pile into a serving dish and serve either warm or cold.

Tip

Quinoa is similar to couscous. It is gluten free and high in protein. Simply make up with water and add vegetables of your choice

Quick Basil Noodles ⓥ

SERVES 4
PER SERVING
249 CALORIES
4G FAT
PREP TIME 5 MINUTES
COOK TIME 10 MINUTES

225g (uncooked weight) noodles
2 leeks, finely sliced
1 garlic clove, crushed
1 red pepper, seeded and sliced
115g mushrooms, sliced
1 tbsp soy sauce
1 tbsp sweet chilli sauce
6 basil leaves, finely shredded

1 Cook the noodles in a pan of boiling water and drain.
2 Heat a non-stick wok. Add the leeks, garlic, red pepper and mushrooms and dry-fry for 2–3 minutes until soft.
3 Add the cooked noodles and the sauces, tossing the ingredients together. Add the basil and mix well.
4 Spoon into serving bowls and serve.

Tip

For extra flavour, add a stock cube to the water when cooking the noodles and save the stock to use in soups and sauces

Vegetable Fried Rice Ⓥ ❄

SERVES 2
PER SERVING
270 CALORIES
3.4G FAT
PREP TIME 10 MINUTES
COOK TIME 20 MINUTES

1 red onion, finely sliced
2 garlic cloves, crushed
1 red pepper, seeded and diced
225g cooked basmati rice
115g frozen peas
115g frozen sweetcorn
1 small red chilli, finely sliced
150ml vegetable stock
salt and freshly ground black pepper
2 tbsps chopped fresh parsley, to garnish

1 Heat a large non-stick pan; add the onion and garlic and
   dry-fry until soft.
2 Add the red pepper and cook for 1
   minute more. Add the rice, peas,
   sweetcorn and chilli. Pour in the
   vegetable stock and cook over a
   high heat until the vegetables are
   hot. Season to taste with salt and
   black pepper.
3 Just before serving sprinkle with the
   chopped fresh parsley.

Tip

For a quick lunch
stir in 1 tbsp
extra light
mayonnaise and
serve cold as a
salad

Baked Cheesy Sweet Potatoes ⓥ

SERVES 4
PER SERVING
186 CALORIES
3.2G FAT
PREP TIME 10 MINUTES
COOK TIME 1 HOUR 10 MINUTES

4 large sweet potatoes
100g Philadelphia Extra Light soft cheese
2 tbsps grated low-fat Cheddar cheese
1 tbsp chopped fresh chives
coarse sea salt

1 Preheat the oven to 200C, 400F, Gas Mark 6.
2 Scrub the sweet potatoes and place in a non-stick roasting
   tin.
3 Sprinkle with sea salt and place in the oven for
   approximately 1 hour until cooked.
4 When cooked, remove from the oven
   and cut in half. Combine the soft
   cheese, Cheddar cheese and chives in
   a small bowl. Spoon into the centre of
   each potato and return to the oven for
   a further 10 minutes until the cheese
   has melted. Serve hot.

Tip

Leaving the skin on potatoes increases their fibre content and gives a nice crispy texture when baking

Tomato and Basil French Bread Pizza Ⓥ

SERVES 2
PER SERVING
180 CALORIES
3.1G FAT
PREP TIME 5 MINUTES
COOK TIME 5 MINUTES

1 × 120g wholemeal baguette
8 fresh basil leaves
4 cherry tomatoes, sliced
28g Philadelphia Extra Light soft cheese

for the tomato sauce
½ small onion, chopped
½ small red pepper
1 × 200g can chopped tomatoes
1 small garlic clove, crushed
a few drops of Worcestershire sauce
salt and freshly ground black pepper to taste

Tip

As a variation sprinkle some dried oregano on top instead of using basil leaves

1 To make the tomato sauce, heat a non-stick frying pan. add the onion and red pepper to the pan and dry-fry until soft. Add the chopped tomatoes, crushed garlic, Worcestershire sauce and seasoning to taste, and simmer gently until the tomatoes have reduced to a thick sauce mixture.
2 Meanwhile, cut the baguette in half and lightly toast. When the tomato sauce mixture is ready, spread on the baguette and top with the basil leaves and cherry tomatoes and then dab small amounts of the soft cheese evenly along the top.
3 Place back under the grill until the mixture is slightly browned.

Desserts

Honey and Ginger Oranges

SERVES 2
PER SERVING
97 CALORIES
0.2G FAT
PREP TIME 5 MINUTES
COOK TIME 20 MINUTES

1 × 2.5cm piece fresh ginger, finely chopped
1 tbsp honey
2 oranges, peeled and sliced

1   Heat the chopped ginger in a pan with the honey and
    1 tbsp boiling water until thick and syrupy.
2   Divide the orange slices between 2 serving bowls and pour
    the syrup over them.

Rocky Road

SERVES 1
75 CALORIES
2.4G FAT
PREP TIME 5 MINUTES

150g low-fat yogurt
5 small marshmallows
a little chocolate sauce for drizzling

1   Place alternate layers of yogurt and marshmallows in a
    glass and drizzle the chocolate sauce on top.

Pineapple and Raspberry Crème

SERVES 4
PER SERVING
67 CALORIES
0.3G FAT
PREP TIME 10 MINUTES

1 small pineapple
115g raspberries
150g 0% fat Greek-style yogurt
zest of 1 orange
sugar to taste (optional)
a few sprigs fresh mint, to decorate

1 Using a sharp, serrated knife, slice off the top and the bottom of the pineapple. Stand the fruit upright and carefully slice away the outer skin in a downward motion, leaving a barrel shape. Slice in half lengthways, then in quarters and across into small chunks and place in a mixing bowl.
2 Add the raspberries, yogurt and orange zest. Sweeten with a little sugar if required and pile into serving glasses. Decorate with fresh mint.

Tip

To choose a fresh, ripe pineapple, give it a little tug at the top. If the leaf comes away easily it is ripe

Pot au Chocolat

SERVES 4
PER SERVING
117 CALORIES
0.6G FAT
PREP TIME 5 MINUTES
COOK TIME 10 MINUTES

1 × 75g packet instant chocolate custard
2 tsps Green & Black's cocoa powder
zest of 1 orange
150g 0% fat Greek-style yogurt
1 tbsp caster sugar
2 egg whites
a few sprigs fresh mint, to decorate

1 Make up the custard with boiling water as per the packet instructions. Stir in the cocoa powder and orange zest, and allow to cool.
2 When cool, fold in the yogurt and caster sugar.
3 Whisk the egg whites until stiff. Carefully fold into the custard mixture, using a metal spoon.
4 Spoon into serving glasses and decorate with fresh mint.

Tip

Vary the flavour by adding a little peppermint essence in place of the orange

Raspberry Panna Cotta

SERVES 6
PER SERVING
129 CALORIES
3.5G FAT
PREP TIME 10 MINUTES
COOK TIME 15 MINUTES

250g fresh raspberries
2 tbsps Silver Spoon Half Spoon sugar
300ml/½ pint semi-skimmed milk
1 vanilla pod
2 tbsps runny honey
4 gelatine leaves, soaked
400g low-fat Greek-style yogurt (3% fat, e.g. Morrisons)
4 mint leaves, to decorate

1   Reserve 4 raspberries for decoration and place the remainder
    in a small saucepan. Add the sugar and 2 tbsps of water.
    Heat gently, mashing the raspberries with a wooden spoon.
    When completely soft, push through a sieve and discard the
    seeds.
2   Heat the milk in a separate pan. Place the vanilla pod on a
    chopping board and, using a small knife, slice lengthways.
    Open the pod and run the knife along the edges to extract
    the vanilla seeds. Add the seeds to the milk.
3   Heat the milk to near boiling, then remove from the heat
    and stir into the raspberry purée.
4   Add the gelatine leaves and whisk well until fully combined.
5   Whisk in the honey and yogurt, then pour into 4 cups or
    dessert moulds. Place in the refrigerator overnight to set.

6 When set, loosen the panna cotta by dipping the cups or moulds very quickly into boiling water, and turn out onto serving plates. Decorate each with a reserved raspberry and a mint leaf.

Tip

You can use disposable plastic cups as moulds for these desserts

Chocolate Banana Fool

SERVES 4
PER SERVING
92 CALORIES
0.6G FAT
PREP TIME 15 MINUTES

1 banana
2 tsps dark brown sugar
2 tsps cocoa powder
300g 0% fat Greek-style yogurt
2 egg whites
1 tsp Silver Spoon Half Spoon sugar
4 mint leaves
8 red berries

Tip

This is a good way of using up very ripe bananas

1 Peel the banana and place in a small bowl with the brown sugar and cocoa powder. Using a fork, mash well together until smooth.
2 Fold in the yogurt.
3 Whisk the egg whites to stiff peaks, using an electric whisk, gradually adding the sugar during the whisking. Carefully fold into the mixture, using a metal spoon.

4 Spoon the mixture into serving glasses. Decorate each
   glass with a mint leaf and 2 red berries.

Sparkling Fresh Fruit Salad

SERVES 4
PER SERVING
149 CALORIES
0.5G FAT
PREP TIME 20 MINUTES

juice of 1 lime
1 eating apple, cored and diced
2 bananas, sliced
1 small melon, chopped
2 oranges, segmented
a few white or red grapes
1 × 1cm piece of stem ginger, finely chopped
300ml/½ pint low-calorie lemonade
fresh mint to decorate

1 Pour the lime juice into a mixing
   bowl. Add the diced apple and sliced
   bananas and toss well, coating the
   fruit to prevent it from discolouring.
2 Add the remaining fruits, then add
   the chopped ginger and mix well.
3 Pour the lemonade over the fruits
   and decorate with fresh mint.

Tip

As a variation, try
replacing the
lemonade with
low-calorie ginger
beer. The salad
tastes just as good
the next day
without the fizz

13

How to Lose Weight Faster

Once you have made a commitment to lose weight, you will want to see fast results. When you can see and feel the rewards for your efforts – your clothes feel looser and you feel healthier – you know the diet is working and you are encouraged to continue.

So what can you do to speed things along a bit and see even greater benefits? Exercise is the key to making this happen. Getting – and then staying – more active on a regular basis will not only speed up your weight-loss progress but it will also help you to stay slim in the long term.

Why exercise is good for you

The health benefits we gain from exercising regularly are now well documented. People who make exercise a habit often tell us how much better they look and feel, how they have never been in better shape and that they have 'found' muscles they didn't know existed. Their skin may have taken on a special glow, radiating good health, and their hair and nails are likely to be in great condition. Overall, they have more energy for life.

These are the real results, the improvements we can actually see and feel. But an effective exercise programme goes a lot deeper than that. It is what happens inside the body that has the biggest life-changing effects and these can not only prolong but, more importantly, improve the quality of your life.

It makes your heart work harder

The heart is a muscle and, if it is not made to work, it will become weaker. The sensation of your heart beating faster when you exert yourself – and that can happen from as normal an activity as going up stairs – shows that you are stimulating the heart muscle and, in turn, making it stronger. Also, when the heart beats faster, you are going to need more air coming into your lungs, so you get another great benefit of making the lungs work hard, which is exactly what they are designed to do!

Finally, as the heart pumps out more blood, the circulatory system (made up of an amazing network of arteries and veins) becomes more efficient at pumping blood and oxygen to every inch of the body, right to the surface of the skin.

For people who want to lose weight, the great result of all this extra activity going on inside the body is that they will be burning lots of extra calories! The longer and more frequently your heart, lungs and circulatory system are made to work hard, the faster you will lose weight.

Tip

Get out of breath every single day for at least 10 minutes

It turns your muscles into fat-burning machines

When you exercise an individual muscle, for instance the biceps when doing a bicep curl or the rectus abdominis when performing an abdominal curl, then that muscle becomes leaner, firmer and stronger. But something else quite important also happens. Within all our muscles are what are called little 'powerhouses' (mitochondria) that multiply considerably in number when a specific muscle is stimulated through exercise. These 'powerhouses' are the centre of the fat-burning process in the body as they are the physical point at which fat is burned off (in the same way that petrol is burned off in your car). Therefore, if you have strong, well-exercised muscles that contain loads of mitochondria, you will be burning body fat efficiently, resulting in a higher metabolism and an ability to lose weight more easily.

Tip

Do a body conditioning workout for all the major muscles of the body at least twice a week

It makes your bones stronger

As we age our bones lose strength but we can slow down that process considerably by doing the right kind of exercise. Swimming, for example, is a great cardiovascular exercise that works the heart and lungs really well but unfortunately has little effect on the bones.

Walking regularly has been proven to keep the thigh and hip bones relatively strong, but to strengthen the bones in the upper body you also need to add some exercises that really load the bones of the wrists, arms and the shoulder area. At the same time if you eat a diet high in calcium you will be doing the very best for your bones.

It keeps your joints mobile

The more active you are, the better your joint health will be. Too sedentary a lifestyle can lead to pain and stiffness in the joints. If you have a condition such as arthritis, it is best to keep moving on a regular basis. Doing some stretching exercises will also ensure that you keep a good range of movement in the joint.

Tip

Do weight-bearing exercises every day. Walking is good for the lower body and 10 press-ups a day will be sufficient for the upper body

 Tip Never sit for long periods. Get up and move around for just 2 minutes every hour and do 10 shoulder rolls

Walk your way to slim hips and thighs

Walking will help keep the hips and thighs in good shape. Our reliance on the car has had a hugely detrimental effect on how much we walk, but we should never underestimate the value of good old-fashioned walking.

Why 10,000 steps a day?

Aiming to walk 10,000 steps per day is the recommended fitness goal. But why this magic number? Will it make us all fitter and slimmer? Will it help us to live longer? The answer is a resounding yes! There is very strong evidence that people who take around 6000 steps per day on average are likely to prolong their lives. And if you do 8–10,000 steps per day regularly you will not only reduce your risk of an early death but you will also promote weight loss. Now that is exactly what we want isn't it!

Use a pedometer

This small piece of equipment can produce BIG changes in your activity levels. Pop it on your waistband for just one day and you will be amazed how much it raises your awareness of your activity levels. It will encourage you to increase your walking so that you can add more to the total! Wear it for a week to find out your total steps for an average day. Fewer than 5000 and you are classed as sedentary. Check out the chart below to see how you score.

Number of steps per day	Activity level
Under 5000	Sedentary lifestyle
5000–7499	Low active
7500–9999	Somewhat active
More than 10,000	Active
More than 12,500	Highly active

How active is your job?

What you do for most of the working day has an enormous bearing on the number of steps you can manage. In a recent survey it was not surprising to find that a postman or woman did the most steps, achieving an average of 15,000 steps per day, and were on their feet for 90 per cent of the time. At the other end of the scale, a lorry driver only managed 2500 steps and spent only five per cent of the day on their feet. Many office workers are shocked to find they only achieve around 2500–3000 steps a day, so 10,000 can seem an impossible target and demotivate some people. And yet increasing the number of steps per day is not as hard as you think.

Take the 'step' approach

So, you find out that you do nowhere near 10,000 steps per day but you want to lose weight and get fitter and healthier. The answer is not to give up but to just set yourself small, achievable goals. Let's say your weekly average is 4200 steps per day. Try adding just another 2000 steps a day by making small changes to your everyday habits. That will take your daily total to more than 6000 steps and you already will be increasing your chances of living longer! Also 2000 steps is about a mile, so let's start adding just a mile to your daily distance.

Ten tips for adding 2000 steps per day
  1 Park further away from your ultimate destination.
  2 Never take the lift or, if it is a very high building, get out three floors down and walk the rest!
  3 If you do use an escalator, walk up it!
  4 At home, never leave items at the bottom of the stairs to take up later. Every trip upstairs adds to your total steps.

continued

5 When talking on the phone, walk around or walk on the spot.

6 When working at a desk, get up and do 50 steps every half hour or so – it only takes 30 seconds.

7 At lunchtime, aim to walk for 20 minutes. That is the equivalent of 2000 steps – a whole mile!

8 Never sit and watch the adverts on TV – they will probably encourage you to eat something anyway. Get up and move around.

9 Change one short car journey to a walking journey – better to use your own fuel than petrol!

10 Meeting a friend to catch up? Make it a 'walking talk' rather than a 'sit and chat'.

Fitness goals for kids

Children should be achieving a lot more steps than adults. They should aim for at least 15,000 steps per day and preferably nearer 20,000. Get them to wear a pedometer and estimate their average steps per day. Then work together as a family to improve both your averages. Encouraging children to have an active lifestyle and being a good role model is one of the best things you can do for their health. At the same time, it can be great fun and provide huge benefits for the whole family.

Ways to be an active family

* Set times aside when you can be active together – aim for twice a week.

* If you have very young children, avoid sitting watching TV with them too often and instead play active games together.

* Pre-teens have a huge physical potential so encourage activities and games with their peers but also try cycling and walking together as a family.

* Teenagers do want more independence, but taking them to the local leisure centre where you can all find an activity to suit is better than sitting in the cinema or a fast food outlet!

How toning exercises shape your hips and thighs

Walking will work your hip and thigh muscles hard, but combining regular walking with a shaping and toning programme will provide the best results.

In particular, our outer and inner thighs are specifically targeted when we perform exercises where those muscles are the prime movers – in other words, when those muscles are doing the majority of the work. If we wanted to specifically target our inner thigh and outer thigh muscles when walking, we would need to walk sideways! The Hip and Thigh Workout in chapter 14 gives you the whole shaping and toning package. And it will also stregthen your bones.

Are you the 'active' type or a 'slouch on the couch'

Your personality does have a bearing on how active you are. Fill in this short fitness questionnaire to find out if you are a naturally active or sedentary person.

1 When you were at school did you . . .?

1 Avoid PE lessons at all costs. ☐

2 Prefer not to do PE but enjoyed it when you did. ☐

3 Generally love all sports and activities and played team games. ☐

2 When you were young and with friends did you . . . ?

1 Sit and chat about your favourite TV programmes. ☐

2 Play outside a lot. ☐

3 Meet up to play sports and try new activities together. ☐

3 With your job do you . . .?

1 Sit at a desk most of the day. ☐

2 Sit at a desk but try to be as active as possible at other times. ☐

3 Spend most of the day doing physical tasks. ☐

4 In your leisure time do you ...?

1 Watch a lot of TV. ☐

2 Get out once or twice a week to do some physical activity. ☐

3 Participate in sports and physical activity three or four times a week. ☐

5 When out shopping would you ...?

1 Always use a lift or escalator rather than the stairs. ☐

2 Occasionally not use the lift/escalator and use the stairs instead. ☐

3 Always take the most active route to the shops. ☐

6 When you have a free day do you prefer to ...?

1 Sit and read. ☐

2 Fit some activity into the day and some relaxation. ☐

3 Take a bike ride or a long walk. ☐

7 When you are on holiday do you prefer to ...?

1 Lie by the pool for two weeks. ☐

2 Mix some active days with relaxation. ☐

3 Fill your days with activity. ☐

continued

8 Do the people you mix with . . .?

    1 Generally 'slouch on the couch'. ☐

    2 Get moving in fits and starts. ☐

    3 Enjoy exercise and do lots of it. ☐

To score

Give yourself 2 points when the number 1 answer was most appropriate.

Give yourself 5 points when the number 2 answer was most appropriate.

Give yourself 10 points if the number 3 answer was most appropriate.

How did you score?

24–39   You have a natural urge to be a 'slouch on the couch'.

40–59   Your fitness is OK but you could probably do more.

60–80   You have a natural urge to be active and probably will always be active.

If you scored low

You do not have a natural urge to move about and have to work harder to lose weight and keep it off. Many sedentary dieters are successful at losing weight initially because they dramatically reduce their food intake. But this is very hard to sustain in the long term and as soon as the food intake creeps back up again then so does the weight.

Top tip for low scorers
Use a pedometer and just add more steps to everyday life – every few steps you take burns an extra calorie! Keep reminding yourself of the value of exercise.

If you scored in the middle of the range
You have real potential for significantly improving your rate of weight loss. The chances are you actually enjoy being more active when you make the effort and you are pleased with the results.

Top tip for middle range scorers
Find an activity or sport you really enjoy and stick with it.

If you scored high
You clearly enjoy being active but may have lost the habit of exercising regularly. Join a gym or go to a regular exercise class to make your weight management more effective. Get into the habit of doing two or three sessions a week.

Top tip for high scorers
If you scored high on activity but are very overweight, then you are eating too much. You probably think that being active alone should keep you slim, but unfortunately that is not the case. Reduce your portions significantly and you will start to lose weight. The combination of eating fewer calories and spending all those extra calories through your new active lifestyle will start to make the weight drop off!

How to increase your willpower for exercise

When we resolve to become more active, we may really mean it at the time, but how many of us succeed? Why is it that some people only last a few days or at the very most a few weeks before they decide that it is not worth the effort? Well, it is a lot to do with the discomfort of making changes to your life and the time it actually takes to make a positive change into a life-long habit.

The most common reasons given for giving up are:

I don't have the time

This is really an excuse, as the recommended guideline of doing 30 minutes of moderate exercise five days a week or 20 minutes of more intense exercise three times a week is certainly do-able for most of us, considering the number of hours we spend watching TV! It all depends how much we want to be more active and if we have the patience to keep at it until the benefits really kick in. Doing the questionnaire on pages 244–6 may have helped you know yourself better.

I hate feeling out of breath

This is not surprising because it is uncomfortable. But feeling slightly breathless and breathing more deeply regularly over a period of time has an amazing effect on how the body functions. Moderate intensity is best and then that awful feeling of fatigue can be avoided. Instead, you feel energised and ready for more!

I'm just too tired to exercise

This is usually a mental tiredness – if you sit at a desk for most of the day, then your tiredness will be blown away when that blood starts pumping round your body and the brain receives the extra oxygen. Regular exercisers always tell you how they feel so much better after an exercise session, particularly after a hard day at the office.

My friend stopped doing it, and then so did I!

This is a difficult one as many of us are certainly more moti-vated by having an exercise buddy to keep us on track. Work on your friend and try to persuade them to keep it up, but if all else fails either look for another, more positive friend or trust your-self to go it alone. When you are looking slim and beautiful, that is the time to visit your friend!

It made my back and joints feel worse!

Then you were doing the wrong type of exercise. With the right guidance from a qualified instructor who understands your condition and an exercise programme that progresses at a very gentle pace, you are less likely to feel worse – only better!

Changing habits

People only make permanent changes in their lives if the bene-fits outweigh the costs. In other words they want to see results, and preferably as quickly as possible. When it comes to losing weight, if you reduce your food intake dramatically you can get results almost instantly and lose several pounds in one week, particularly if you have a lot of weight to lose.

Results from exercise do take slightly longer, but if you give yourself just one month, the effects of a consistent exercise programme will really start to show. By then, regular exercise will have become a habit and you will be less likely to give it up. Make this the right time for you!

Top tips for making exercise a habit

* Find an activity you like doing – that is the most important step to encourage you to keep it up.
* Plan a realistic schedule of activity – two or three times a week may be sufficient.
* Find a friend who wants to achieve the same results as you and arrange to meet at the same time every week.
* Wear a pedometer.
* Always have exercise kit handy (e.g. in the car).
* Mix with active people.
* Think positive. This really does help you to make permanent changes to your life.
* Make it fun!

So if you want to lose weight faster, make regular exercise as much a part of your lifestyle as eating low-fat, low-Gi foods. In the end you will have a great-looking body to prove that it was all worthwhile.

Slim Hips and Thighs in Super-Quick Time!

This highly effective toning programme targets the inner and outer thighs as well as the gluteal (buttock) muscles to give you slim hips and shapely thighs – fast.

How to use this programme

* You can do this programme every day if you want but aim to do it at least three times per week to see real results.
* There are two levels. If you are new to exercise, then start with the Level 1 exercises before progressing to Level 2.
* There are only six exercises for each level, so your workout will take no more than 10 minutes.
* Most of the exercises for Level 2 require a resistance band. This adds more weight to each exercise, which gives quicker results, so it is definitely worth buying one.

Safety tips

* Always do the warm-up exercises at the start of the programme. They loosen the joints and increase circulation to prepare you fully for the main programme.
* Wear loose and comfortable clothing.
* Drink water regularly to keep well hydrated.
* Breathe regularly and evenly through each exercise. Always breathe out on the effort (the lifting part of the movement) and in as you lower.
* Always do the stretches at the end of the programme. They will return the muscles to their original length, reduce stiffness and help you stay flexible.

Warm-up moves

1 March on spot
Stand tall and march on the spot, making sure the whole foot makes contact with the floor on each step. Let the arms swing naturally. Do 50 steps between each of the warm-up moves that follow.

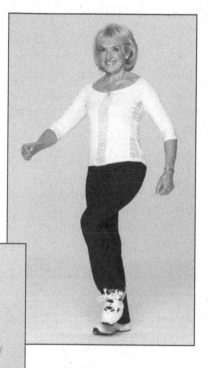

2 Hip circling
Take your feet wider than shoulder width, with knees slightly bent, and circle your hips 10 times clockwise and 10 times anti-clockwise. Try to keep your upper body still and hold your tummy in tight.

3 Knee bends

Stand with feet slightly turned out and wider than hip width. Bend from the hips and knees, taking your hips back as if about to sit in a chair. Keep your knees in line with your feet, your back straight and your head looking forward. Lift again without locking the knees. Do 10 times slowly.

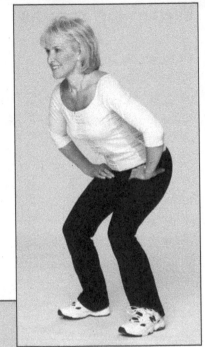

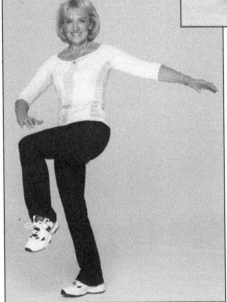

4 Knee lifts

Stand upright with feet together. Lift alternate knees to hip height, taking the opposite hand towards the opposite knee. Keep your back straight and head up. Change legs for 16 repetitions.

The hip and thigh workout

Level 1

1 Thigh shaper

Stand upright in front of a sturdy chair, with feet parallel and hands on hips (a). Pull your tummy in, push your hips back and bend your knees as if about to sit on the chair (b).

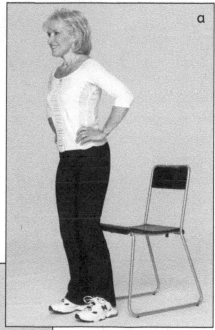

Keep your back straight and your knees in line with your toes. Then come up again, taking care not to lock out the knees as you lift, and look straight ahead. Do 10 repetitions, then rest and do another set.

2 Inner thigh tightener

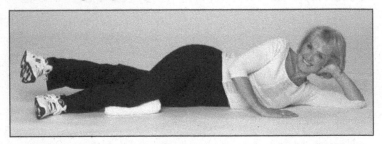

Lie on your side with your head supported in your hand. Rest your other hand on the floor in front. Bend the top knee and place it on a rolled-up towel to bring the hip in line, and straighten the underneath leg. Now, keeping that leg straight, toes pulling towards you and heel pushing away, lift and lower it with control. Do 10 repetitions, then rest and repeat. Repeat on the other side.

3 Hip toner

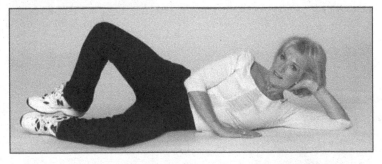

Lie on your side and bend both knees at a 45-degree angle, with feet in line with your hips. Now, keeping your hips stacked and your feet firmly pressing together, lift the top knee away from the bottom knee, and then lower again. Breathe out as you lift and in as you lower. Do 10 repetitions, then rest and do another set. Repeat on the other side.

4 Bottom shaper

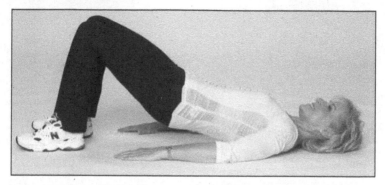

Lie on your back with knees bent and feet flat on the floor hip-width apart and close to your hips. Keeping your upper body relaxed, lift your hips without arching your back, and then lower again. Lift and lower 10 times, keeping the movement smooth and controlled.

5 Outer thigh toner

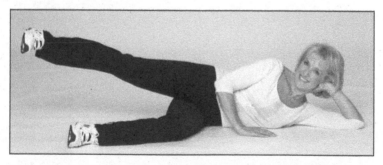

Lie on your side with your underneath leg bent at a 90-degree angle and the top leg out straight in line with the hip. Pull the toes of the top foot towards you and press the heel away. Pull your tummy in to hold your trunk still and lift the top leg to just above hip height, and then lower again. Do 10 repetitions, then rest and do another set. Repeat on the other side.

6 Bottom tightener

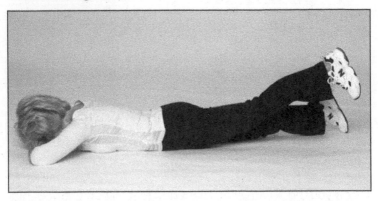

Lie on your front with your head resting on your hands and both legs just wider than hip width. Slowly lift alternate legs no higher than the length of your foot and try to push the hip of the raised leg away from you as you lift. Keep both hips facing the floor and your upper body relaxed. Repeat 10 times (5 each leg), and then rest and do another set.

The hip and thigh workout

Level 2

1 Thigh shaper with band

Stand in front of a sturdy chair with both feet on the centre of a resistance band. Grip the ends of the band between the thumb and forefinger (a). Pull the band up to hip height (or to waist height to make it harder)

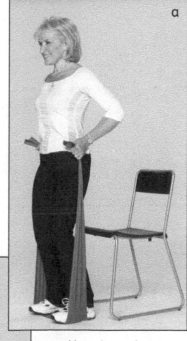

and bend your knees and hips, pushing your hips back as if about to sit on the chair (b). Then fix your feet firmly on the floor as you straighten your legs without locking the knees at the top. Repeat 10 times, then rest and do another set.

2 Inner thigh tightener with chair

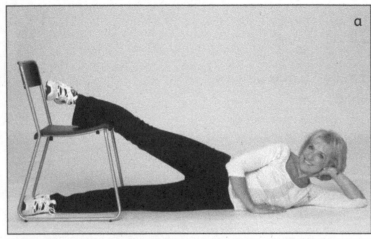

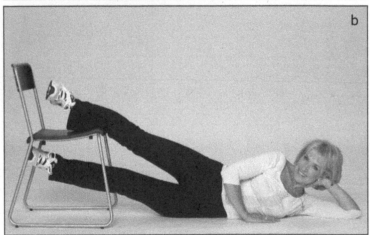

Lie on your side with your top leg on the chair seat and your bottom leg extended on the floor underneath. Both legs should be in line with your trunk (a). Now, keeping your bottom leg straight, lift it under the seat (b), and lower again. Lift and lower for 10 repetitions, then rest and do another set. Repeat on the other side.

3 Hip toner

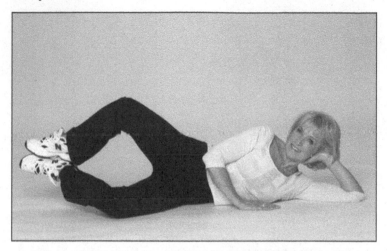

Lie on your side with both legs bent at a 45-degree angle and feet in line with your hips. Pull your tummy in to support your back and, keeping both feet together, lift the top knee away from the bottom knee. Now lift both feet off the floor, still keeping the feet firmly together. Make sure your hips stay stacked on top of each other and do not let them drop back. Lower again and repeat. Do 8 slow and controlled repetitions, and then repeat on the other side.

4 Bottom shaper with band

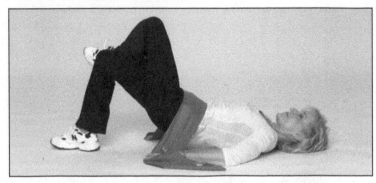

Lie on your back with knees bent and feet flat on the floor, close to your hips. Drape the band across your hips and secure it on the floor with your palms. Place one ankle on top of the opposite knee. Now lift your hips off the floor without arching your back. Lower again under control. Do 10 repetitions, then rest and do another set.

5 Outer thigh toner with band

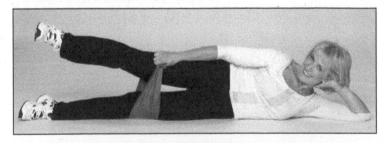

Wrap the band around your lower thighs, just above the knees, and secure the ends firmly in your right hand. Now lie on your left side, with your body in a straight line and hips stacked on top of each other. Lift and lower the top leg slowly, feeling the resistance of the band. Do 10 repetitions, and then rest and do another set. Repeat on the other side.

6 Bottom tightener

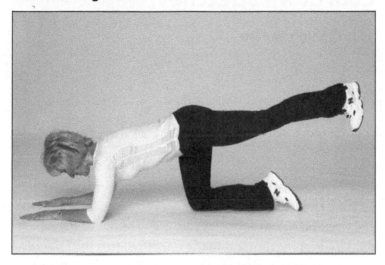

Come up onto your elbows and knees, with elbows directly under your shoulders and knees under hips. Extend your right leg out, with toes in contact with the floor. Keep your hips facing the floor and your tummy pulled in. Now lift and lower one leg, leading with the heel and only lifting to hip height. Do 10 repetitions, then change legs. Then do another set on each leg.

Cool down stretches

1 Front thigh stretch

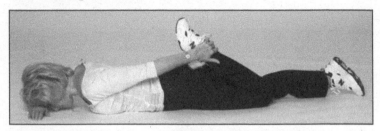

Lie on your front and rest your head on your right hand. Bend your left knee and hold the ankle with your left hand. Keeping your hips facing the floor and your knees together, gently press your left hip firmly into the floor to stretch the front of the hip as well as the front of the thigh. Hold for 10 seconds, then change legs and repeat.

2 Bottom stretch

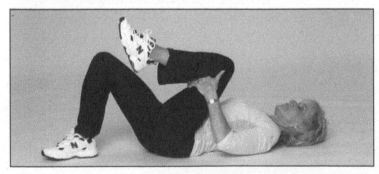

Lie on your back with knees bent, and then bring your left leg up to hold behind the left thigh. Keep both hips square on the floor and pull the left knee closer to your chest to feel a stretch in the back of the left hip. Hold for 10 seconds, and then do the next stretch before changing legs.

3 Back thigh stretch

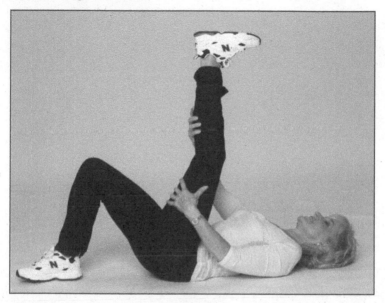

Straighten your left leg and hold around the back of the calf and the back of the thigh. Try to straighten the leg as much as possible but keep both hips on the floor. Hold for 10 seconds, then take a deep breath and, as you breathe out, straighten the leg further to develop the stretch. Hold for 10 seconds more. Now do stretches 2 and 3 on the other leg.

4 Inner thigh stretch

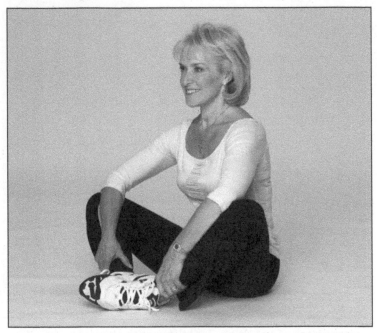

Sit up straight with soles of the feet together and hold both ankles. Keeping your back straight and head up, press your elbows on the insides of your knees to push your knees towards the floor. Hold for 10 seconds, then take a breath in and, as you breathe out, press harder on the insides of the knees for a further 10 seconds.

5 Outer thigh stretch

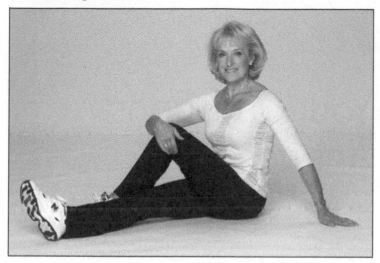

Sit upright with both legs out in front, and then take your left leg across your right knee, placing your left foot flat on the floor. Place your right hand around the outside of your left knee and rest your left hand on the floor. Now draw the left knee further across your chest to feel a stretch in the left hip. Hold for 10 seconds, then change legs and repeat.

15

Your Questions Answered

Each week I receive a big postbag of letters from readers who want to lose weight or from slimmers who have already started a weight-loss plan and need further advice. Here's a selection of typical questions.

Q *Is tuna an oily fish and does it count as one of the recommended portions of oily fish per week?*

A Tuna is not an oily fish but is still very good for us, so it is fine to eat it whenever you like. Try to buy tuna canned in brine or plain water in preference to oil to keep the calories and fat down. Oily fish includes salmon, herring, mackerel, sardines and pilchards. Try to have one or two portions of one of these each week to be sure of getting your essential fatty acids and to help keep your heart healthy.

Q *Are sweet potatoes a good substitute for old potatoes? Do they have the same number of calories?*

A Despite their somewhat unattractive appearance, sweet potatoes taste fabulous and are enjoying a huge rise in popularity because of the greater awareness of low-Gi eating. Sweet potatoes are low Gi (that's good) while old, regular potatoes are high Gi (not so good). The reason for these different Gi ratings is that sweet potatoes take longer to digest, which means they release their energy more slowly and this keeps our blood sugar levels more constant.

Old potatoes are digested more quickly, because of their age, and so they release energy more rapidly, resulting in faster fluctuations in our blood sugar levels. You can, however, slow down their digestion by eating an old baked potato with a low-Gi topping such as baked beans. You can bake a sweet potato in the oven in the same way as baking an old one (although for a shorter time as sweet potatoes cook more swiftly) and top it with baked beans or some other healthy topping. You can also eat the skin as this contains valuable fibre.

Old potatoes offer 75 calories per 100g and sweet potatoes 86 calories per 100g. More, I know, but they are better for you and they taste delicious.

Q *I am one of your male dieters and I try to stay in reasonable shape by eating healthily. Recently I have not been as active as I usually am and, while my clothes are feeling a little tighter, my weight hasn't changed on the scales. Why is this?*

A It is the lack of exercise that is the culprit here. When you exercise regularly, you burn fat and tone your muscles and this makes you slimmer, particularly around the trunk. If you stop your regular activity for any length of time you will lose some of that muscle tone and a little extra fat will creep on in its place. Your body composition will change and you will store some excess fat around your middle. Just start exercising again and you will soon lose those extra inches.

Q *Is it true that a good night's sleep can help you lose weight?*

A Yes it is and it's to do with our hormones, especially one called 'cortisol'. When we are deprived of sleep, we release cortisol at an increased level and this makes us feel hungry, even if we have had sufficient to eat. People who lose sleep on a regular basis will tend to feel hungrier than people with regular sleep patterns. At the same time, they will feel tired and won't have much energy to be very active, which means they will end up burning fewer calories than someone who is rested and more energetic.

Q *I visit family and friends a lot at weekends. How can I avoid eating high-fat foods without offending them?*

A Many of us find weekends difficult because we are out of our usual working-week-routine where time pressures dictate what and when we eat. When visiting friends it becomes a celebration and much thought will have been put into planning the meals. Why not tell your friends you are trying really hard to lose a few pounds at the moment and, while you can eat anything in principle, you are trying to eat less fat – and that includes avoiding olive oil. Enthuse about how much weight you have lost so far and how much better you feel and I am sure they will support and encourage you by feeding you thoughtfully.

Q *I've been dieting for a few months and done really well but now I have come to a standstill and haven't lost any weight for the last three weeks. Why is that?*

A What you are experiencing is not uncommon and is often referred to as 'reaching a plateau'. There are various reasons for this but you can certainly start losing weight again if you do the following.

Are you still using your portion pots? Just for a week measure or weigh out your portions, as it is easy to start eating a little more than you did at the beginning of the diet without realising it.

Are you as physically active now as you were at the beginning of your diet? Even if you are, try to do a bit extra aerobic exercise anyway as this will speed up your metabolism as well as burn extra calories and fat. Then try changing some of your regular menu items such as your regular breakfast cereal or lunch for something different. It will bring freshness and variety to your dieting efforts and may help to keep you focused.

Also, take the time to measure yourself. Sometimes we lose inches and this can be a great encouragement when the scales seem to stick.

Q *My scales broke and I bought some new ones yesterday but, according to these, I seem to have gained weight. Is it common for scales to vary?*

A Unless you buy professional scales, such as the ones we use at Rosemary Conley classes, you are unlikely to get a totally accurate reading. However, domestic ones should still indicate your progress if you weigh yourself weekly. It's not a problem if they indicate you weigh a pound or two more or less than you really are. What matters if you are trying to lose weight is that you can see the reading going down. For accuracy, avoid keeping scales in a damp room such as the bathroom, place them on a hard and level surface (not carpet) or on a wooden board. Try not to become a slave to the scales and, for the most accurate results, weigh yourself only once a week, at the same time of day each week and in the same clothes (or none at all).

Q *Why is it so important to drink water during a workout?*

A It's all about dehydration. We lose water all the time but during exercise we lose much more than usual and we can quickly become dehydrated. If our muscles become dehydrated, they don't work so well and we also find our energy levels falling. In trials it was discovered that drinking a little and often throughout a workout helps people keep going for much longer. We should all be drinking a couple of litres of water a day anyway, but on the days that we exercise we should try to drink even more.

Q *Is it true that if I build up my muscles I will burn fat faster?*

A Yes. Our muscles are fat-burning factories, so it follows that the bigger and stronger they are, the more fat they will burn. It is estimated that for every extra pound of muscle that we have, we will burn around an extra 35 calories a day. Of course muscles take time to build and grow, but doing muscle-strengthening exercises regularly, say three times a week, using weights or a resistance band, will help you to build your muscle size and strength and make you a faster fat-burner as well as improving your body shape.

Q *Should I eat before or after exercising?*

A It all depends on when you ate last. If you eat three good meals a day it may not be necessary to eat before your workout, but if you haven't eaten for, say, five hours and you go straight to a class or to the gym from work, I recommend you eat a light, low-Gi snack beforehand. A banana or a small sandwich made with wholegrain bread are both good options.

Avoid fatty foods, but drink plenty of water. Aim to eat within 90 minutes of completing your workout to ensure you replace the glycogen stores in your muscles. Eating a carbohydrate-based snack with some low-fat protein such as chicken is ideal.

Q *I don't always have time to cook proper meals. Are supermarket ready meals OK to eat when dieting?*

A Ready meals vary, so check the labels to find out the fat and calorie content and what ingredients they contain. Even better, why not add ready-made stir-fry sauces to fresh ingredients? This is still a quick way of preparing meals but much healthier and you have more control of the food content. For example, dry-fry some chicken pieces in a non-stick wok until almost cooked, add some chopped peppers, onion, celery and mushrooms and then stir in the sauce. Serve with basmati rice or pasta for a delicious, nutritious meal.

Q *You always tell us to drink plenty of water. Does tea count towards my water intake?*

A Yes, it does. Tea is now recognised as a hydrating, healthy drink and can contribute to our daily fluid intake. It also contains antioxidants that help boost our immune system. If you drink it with milk, use milk from your daily allowance and then you don't need to count the calories as extra as they are already included in your daily total. Of course, if you take sugar, you will need to take into account the additional calories from that.

Q *I want to lose weight but I don't want to give up alcohol. Do I have to?*

A No, but you may have to moderate your intake. I believe it is really important to make a diet work by including the things we really enjoy, otherwise our willpower will be overstretched and in a weak moment we may throw in the towel and go on a binge!

For good health, women should restrict their weekly alcohol intake to 14 units a week and men to 21. A unit is a small glass of wine or 300ml/½ pint of regular (not strong) lager or beer, or a single shot of spirits. So, you could have two units a day and count the calories into your daily total.

In round figures, a small glass of wine is around 100 calories, as is 300ml/½ pint of beer, while a single measure of spirit (gin, whisky, brandy, vodka or rum) is about 50 calories. If you use slimline mixers, you can avoid adding extra calories.

Q *My aerobics instructor says that doing arm movements with the exercises will burn extra calories. Is that right?*

A It certainly is! When we exercise aerobically we become slightly breathless as the body requires more oxygen to cope with the activity. Oxygen enters our bloodstream through our lungs and is pumped around the body by the heart, supplying energy to the muscles. Using arm movements increases the intensity of the exercise, which means we burn more calories during our exercise session.

Q *I've heard that hydrogenated fats are bad for us but what actually are they?*

A During the manufacturing process, pure vegetable oils have hydrogen bubbled through them to improve their texture, flavour and shelf-life, resulting in a more solid fat which goes on to be used in many processed foods such as cakes, pastries, biscuits, ready meals and take-aways. This hydrogenation process alters the texture and also the way that the oils act in the body. They can become as much of a health risk as eating saturated fats such as lard or butter and are definitely something to avoid – both for your health and for your waistline.

Q *I am overweight but I have a flat, shapeless bottom. Can you suggest some exercises to give me a better shape?*

A We all have different body shapes and you can blame your genes for your flattish backside. The good news is that we can increase the size of the gluteal (buttock) muscle through exercise. Going up and down stairs is a simple but effective way to tone it; using a stepping machine is another.

Try the bottom tightener exercise on page 263. Also try standing behind a chair and, keeping your hips facing the front without twisting them, lift alternate legs behind you with toes pointing forward and not out. Practise this 12 times twice a day and you will see an improvement to your shape within about a month or two.

Q *I was determined to lose weight this year and tried hard to stop eating chocolate. I have lost a stone and a half already but my craving for chocolate is as great as ever. Any tips?*

A Losing more than 20lb, as you have done, is a real achievement and will have significantly improved your health. If chocolate is so important to you, there are ways of incorporating it into your diet, providing you can trust yourself not to have a chocolate binge once you get the taste! Try my Low Fat Belgian Chocolate Mousse, which is available from most supermarkets. You can even freeze it and eat it like ice cream. Allowing yourself one a day will give you a significant chocolate 'fix' without doing any damage to your diet but make sure you count the 118 calories it contains into your daily allowance.

Q *How quickly can I lose 2 stone? I have just been invited to join friends for a fabulous holiday in three months' time and I want to look good on the beach. What is a realistic goal to aim for?*

A We all respond to goals and deadlines, so see this as a golden opportunity to focus on your weight-loss campaign. If you stick to the Fat Attack Fortnight diet in this book for two weeks and then increase the calories to 1400 a day thereafter and also do some form of aerobic (fat-burning) activity on five days a week for about 30 minutes, you could lose your excess 2 stone by the time you go away. Carry a picture of your holiday location in your handbag to keep reminding yourself of your goal. Try to do some toning exercises too to improve your body shape as you slim down.

Q *I'm getting bored with my sandwich packed lunches. Any ideas for something that's a bit different for me to eat in the car as I travel between clients?*

A It's easy to ring the changes from sandwiches by making home-made wraps. Spread a wholemeal tortilla with spicy dipping sauce and then add chopped peppers, celery, cucumber, red onion and some wafer thin ham or tuna. Roll up the tortilla, tucking in the sides as you go, and keep it all in one – rather than cutting it in half – and it will travel well.

Another healthy option is to chop up lots of different salad vegetables, like sweetcorn, carrots, raw cauliflower florets, spring onions, celery, red onion, peppers, cucumber and half a red chilli, into tiny pieces and mix with 50 grams of cold, boiled pasta. Then toss it all together with some oil-free dressing and freshly ground black pepper and pack it in a plastic container with a lid. Keep it cool and it will stay fresh and it is easy to eat with a fork.

Q *I have to admit I hate aerobic exercise. Can I lose weight without working out?*

A Lots of people don't like exercising aerobically, which involves increasing your heart rate and getting a bit warm and breathless. When I was researching my Gi Jeans Diet I asked my trial team whether or not they enjoyed exercising; first, when they started, and then, how they felt after following the diet and fitness programme for the eight-week trial. A large number admitted to 'hating' exercise at the beginning but almost 90 per cent of them changed their view by the end and said they 'really enjoyed it now'!

I think some people don't like the 'thought' of exercising – having to change into fitness wear, feeling hot and sweaty afterwards, wearing figure-hugging clothing when we don't feel confident about our bodies – but once we've done it we feel great! Apart from the release of endorphins (happy hormones) during our workout, the feeling of satisfaction when we've actually done it is tremendous. And that's before we've enjoyed the invisible benefits to our health and wellbeing: it exercises our heart and lungs so that we become much fitter physically; it carries more oxygen around our bodies which helps our skin to shrink back as we lose weight; it keeps our joints and muscles active, which helps us to stay in shape.

The key is to find a form of aerobic exercise that you enjoy. If you're frightened that you won't cope in a class, get yourself a fitness DVD and practise at home first to familiarise yourself with some of the moves.

Q *We hear so often that we should eat five portions of fruit and vegetables daily. Does that mean five portions of fruit and five of vegetables, or a total of five portions?*

A Fruit and vegetables are essential for good health and we should eat a minimum of five portions in total daily. It doesn't matter if they are all fruit or all vegetables. It is down to personal preference and aiming for five-a-day is a great starting point.

16

Staying Slim

Losing weight is a real learning experience, but maintaining your new weight in the long term can be more of a challenge.

Following a weight-reducing plan is an interesting and rewarding journey. Discovering which foods are high in fat and calories can be a real eye-opener. Then there's the challenge of learning how to cook the low-fat way and the discipline of making time to exercise.

At the end of each week, when we step on the scales and see how many pounds we have lost, we feel it has all been worth the effort and are motivated to take up the challenge for the next seven days. And then we are rewarded all over again! It just gets better as we begin to feel our clothes getting looser and we can buy new ones in sizes that we haven't worn for years!

Getting to goal

Once we reach our goal weight, we can't believe that we have actually 'done it'. All those weeks and months of saying 'no' to that chocolate, refusing that piece of cake, ordering a jacket potato instead of chips, going for our power walk in the rain seem worthwhile! Now we are wearing our size 10 or 12 dress or jeans and we lap up the compliments from people we haven't seen in months.

But what next? Reaching our goal is really exciting, but maintaining it is, well, fairly uneventful. And that's true. But, hey, you've actually achieved what you set out to and you need to recognise the monumental achievement that you have pulled off! Can you imagine how many people would love to be at their goal weight! With almost 60 per cent of the UK population being overweight or obese and suffering health problems as a result, you are now in that special, elite, healthy, fit, enviable section of the population who is SLIM! Yes! You are officially SLIM!

So, what do you do NOW to keep that way? Try these ten tips to help you stay on track.

Ten tips for successful weight maintenance

1 Set yourself some new goals. Why not take up a lifelong dream challenge such as walking the Great Wall of China, parachuting out of an aeroplane or running the London Marathon and raising money for your favourite charity? Such a challenge will give you the motivation to keep exercising, which will help keep you slim!

2 Take all your 'big' clothes to the charity shop – except for your very largest garment, which you should keep as a memento of your achievements.

3 Make a conscious effort NOT to slip back into your old eating habits such as spreading butter on your bread or eating a bar of chocolate mid-morning at work. Keep on eating and cooking the low-fat way. It should become your normal way of life – for ever.

4 Remember that you are not actually 'dieting' now, so if it's someone's birthday and it's cream cakes all round, have one. Thoroughly enjoy it and appreciate it as a treat.

5 Stay active. Keep attending your class every week as the workout will keep you fit and in good shape and you can pop on the scales to check your weight maintenance.

6 Now that you've reached your goal weight you may be tempted to think you can go back to indulging as you used to. If you start eating or drinking too much again, the weight will pile back on in no time. Remember, it's much harder to lose it the second time around, so don't be tempted!

7 Enjoy being fit and slim. Enjoy buying new clothes. Enjoy feeling your flat stomach when you lie in bed. Enjoy running around with your children and appreciate your feeling of 'lightness'. Enjoy the compliments from your husband or partner when they put their arms around your waist and comment on how slim you feel.

8 Chill out about food and calories. That isn't a licence to eat anything and everything you see but it is important for you to learn to train your brain away from food so that you are not a slave to food any more. You CAN do this.

9 Take a photograph of yourself looking your best. Appreciate how far you have come to reach this

continued

point and keep that photograph handy, together with your 'before' picture, to remind you of your achievement.

10 Avoid stepping on the scales every day. You will know from the way your clothes fit whether you have gained or lost weight. Scales can motivate and de-motivate. If you have lost weight you can be tempted to eat more 'because you are in credit'. If you've gained a pound you can go into panic mode and find yourself stressed and diving for your 'weakest-link' food such as biscuits, chocolate, or crisps. So if your clothes start feeling tight, eat a bit less and do a bit more activity for about three days and the inches will disappear. Do you want to be slim more than you want to eat that chocolate bar? Yes, of course you do!

Portion Pots

Food	Pot	Weight	Kcal
Beans and pulses			
Baked beans	yellow	115g	84 kcal
Lentils (cooked)	yellow	165g	175 kcal
Lentils (uncooked)	blue	50g	175 kcal
Breakfast cereals			
All-Bran	yellow	30g	84 kcal
All-Bran	red	60g	168 kcal
Bran flakes	red	50g	163 kcal
Fruit 'n Fibre	red	50g	183 kcal
Muesli	yellow	50g	183 kcal
Muesli	blue	40g	146 kcal
Porridge (cooked in water)	yellow	122g	125 kcal
Porridge oats (uncooked)	blue	35g	125 kcal
Special K	green	50g	187 kcal
Special K	red	40g	150 kcal
Special K	yellow	20g	75 kcal
Sugar Puffs	green	40g	152 kcal
Sugar Puffs	red	30g	114 kcal
Sultana Bran	yellow	25g	80 kcal
Sultana Bran	red	50g	159 kcal
Cheese			
Cheddar, grated (low fat)	blue	20g	82 kcal
Cottage cheese (low fat)	blue	100g	98 kcal

Food	Pot	Weight	Kcal
Coleslaw			
Coleslaw (low calorie)	blue	85g	78 kcal
Couscous			
Couscous (cooked)	red	107g	185 kcal
Couscous (uncooked)	blue	50g	185 kcal
Fromage frais			
Fromage frais	blue	85g	46 kcal
Fromage frais	yellow	135g	73 kcal
Fruit and fruit juice			
Blueberries	yellow	70g	38 kcal
Fruit juice	yellow	125ml	63 kcal
Raspberries	red	115g	29 kcal
Oats			
Porridge (cooked in water)	yellow	122g	125 kcal
Porridge oats (uncooked)	blue	35g	125 kcal
Pasta			
Pasta shapes (cooked)	green	176g	280 kcal
Pasta shapes (cooked)	red	110g	175 kcal
Pasta shapes (uncooked)	red	80g	280 kcal
Pasta shapes (uncooked)	yellow	45g	175 kcal
Potatoes			
Potato (mashed)	red	200g	172 kcal
Potato (mashed)	yellow	100g	86 kcal

Food	Pot	Weight	Kcal
Sweet potato (mashed)	red	250g	210 kcal
Sweet potato (mashed)	yellow	100g	84 kcal

Rice and noodles

Basmati rice (cooked)	red	144g	205 kcal
Basmati rice (uncooked)	blue	55g	205 kcal
Noodles, egg (cooked) (equivalent to 1 × 65g block uncooked)	green	170g	225 kcal

Sauces

Tomato salsa	blue	75g	23 kcal

Vegetables

Peas (frozen)	yellow	70g	40 kcal

Wine

Wine	yellow	125ml	88 kcal

Yogurt

Yogurt (0% fat Greek-style)	blue	80g	42 kcal
Yogurt (low fat)	blue	80g	72 kcal

Portion Pot sizes/volume

blue	80ml
yellow	125ml
red	250ml
green	330ml

Basal Metabolic Rate (BMR) Table

| Women aged 18–29 | | | Women aged 30–59 | | | Women aged 60–74 | | |
| Body Weight | | | Body Weight | | | Body Weight | | |
Stones	Kilos	BMR	Stones	Kilos	BMR	Stones	Kilos	BMR
7	45	1147	7	45	1208	7	45	1048
7.5	48	1194	7.5	48	1233	7.5	48	1073
8	51	1241	8	51	1259	8	51	1099
8.5	54	1288	8.5	54	1285	8.5	54	1125
9	57	1335	9	57	1311	9	57	1151
9.5	60.5	1382	9.5	60.5	1337	9.5	60.5	1176
10	64	1430	10	64	1373	10	64	1202
10.5	67	1477	10.5	67	1389	10.5	67	1228
11	70	1524	11	70	1414	11	70	1254
11.5	73	1571	11.5	73	1440	11.5	73	1279
12	76	1618	12	76	1466	12	76	1305
12.5	80	1665	12.5	80	1492	12.5	80	1331

13	83	1712	13	83	1518	13	83	1357
13.5	86	1760	13.5	86	1544	13.5	86	1382
14	89	1807	14	89	1570	14	89	1408
14.5	92	1854	14.5	92	1595	14.5	92	1434
15	95.5	1901	15	95.5	1621	15	95.5	1460
15.5	99	1948	15.5	99	1647	15.5	99	1485
16	102	1995	16	102	1673	16	102	1511
16.5	105	2043	16.5	105	1699	16.5	105	1537
17	108	2090	17	108	1725	17	108	1563
17.5	111	2137	17.5	111	1751	17.5	111	1588
18	115	2184	18	115	1776	18	115	1614
18.5	118	2231	18.5	118	1802	18.5	118	1640
19	121	2278	19	121	1828	19	121	1666
19.5	124	2325	19.5	124	1854	19.5	124	1691
20	127	2373	20	127	1880	20	127	1717

Basal Metabolic Rate (BMR) Table

| Men aged 18–29 | | | Men aged 30–59 | | | Men aged 60–74 | | |
| Body Weight | | | Body Weight | | | Body Weight | | |
Stones	Kilos	BMR	Stones	Kilos	BMR	Stones	Kilos	BMR
7	45	1363	7	45	1384	7	45	1232
7.5	48	1411	7.5	48	1421	7.5	48	1270
8	51	1459	8	51	1457	8	51	1307
8.5	54	1507	8.5	54	1494	8.5	54	1345
9	57	1555	9	57	1530	9	57	1383
9.5	60.5	1602	9.5	60.5	1567	9.5	60.5	1421
10	64	1650	10	64	1603	10	64	1459
10.5	67	1698	10.5	67	1640	10.5	67	1497
11	70	1746	11	70	1676	11	70	1535
11.5	73	1794	11.5	73	1713	11.5	73	1573
12	76	1842	12	76	1749	12	76	1611
12.5	80	1890	12.5	80	1786	12.5	80	1649

13	83	1938	13	83	1822	13	83	1687
13.5	86	1986	13.5	86	1859	13.5	86	1725
14	89	2034	14	89	1895	14	89	1763
14.5	92	2082	14.5	92	1932	14.5	92	1801
15	95.5	2129	15	95.5	1968	15	95.5	1839
15.5	99	2177	15.5	99	2005	15.5	99	1877
16	102	2225	16	102	2041	16	102	1915
16.5	105	2273	16.5	105	2078	16.5	105	1953
17	108	2321	17	108	2114	17	108	1991
17.5	111	2369	17.5	111	2151	17.5	111	2028
18	115	2417	18	115	2187	18	115	2066
18.5	118	2465	18.5	118	2224	18.5	118	2104
19	121	2513	19	121	2260	19	121	2142
19.5	124	2561	19.5	124	2297	19.5	124	2180
20	127	2609	20	127	2333	20	127	2218

Weight-loss progress chart

	WEIGHT NOW	POUNDS/KG LOST	TOTAL LOSS TO DATE
Start day Date:			
Week 1 Date:			
Week 2 Date:			
Week 3 Date:			
Week 4 Date:			
Week 5 Date:			
Week 6 Date:			
Week 7 Date:			
Week 8 Date:			
Week 9 Date:			
Week 10 Date:			
Week 11 Date:			
Week 12 Date:			

	WEIGHT NOW	POUNDS/KG LOST	TOTAL LOSS TO DATE
Week 13 Date:			
Week 14 Date:			
Week 15 Date:			
Week 16 Date:			
Week 17 Date:			
Week 18 Date:			
Week 19 Date:			
Week 20 Date:			
Week 21 Date:			
Week 22 Date:			
Week 23 Date:			
Week 24 Date:			

Weight-loss graph

Make up your own graph for each stone you lose, following the example below.

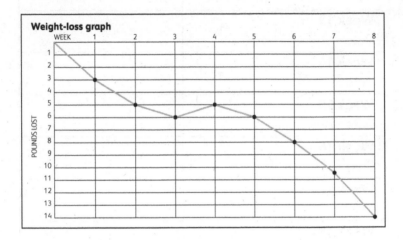

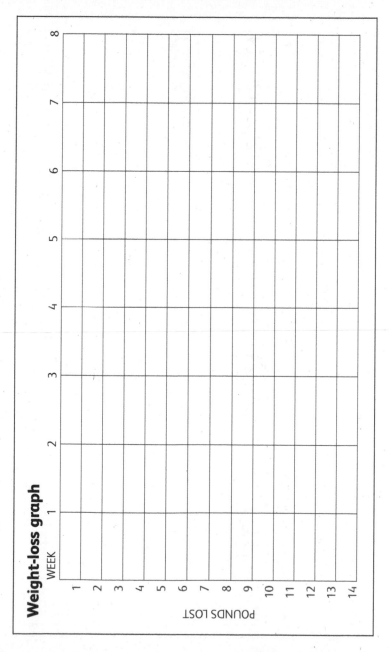

Weight-loss graph

WEEK

POUNDS LOST

Inches/centimetre accumulator

| 1 | 2 | 3 | 4 | 5 | 6 | 7 | 8 | 9 | 10 | 11 | 12 | 13 | 14 | 15 | 16 | 17 |

You can tick or colour the relevant number of inches lost – as you lose them

| 18 |

| 19 | 20 | 21 | 22 | 23 | 24 | 25 | 26 | 27 | 28 | 29 | 30 | 31 | 32 | 33 | 34 | 35 |

| 36 |

| 37 | 38 | 39 | 40 | 41 | 42 | 43 | 44 | 45 | 46 | 47 | 48 | 49 | 50 | 51 | 52 | 53 |

| 54 |

| 55 | 56 | 57 | 58 | 59 | 60 | 61 | 62 | 63 | 64 | 65 | 66 | 67 | 68 | 69 | 70 | 71 |

| 72 |

| 73 | 74 | 75 | 76 | 77 | 78 | 79 | 80 | 81 | 82 | 83 | 84 | 85 | 86 | 87 | 88 | 89 |

How to measure yourself

Take the time to measure yourself once a week. It will provide the most encouraging proof of your progress, as sometimes we lose inches or centimetres when the scales are 'sticking'. Enter your measurements on the chart on page 298.

Widest measurement around the bust

Smallest measurement around the upper arm

Smallest measurement around the waist

Widest measurement around the hips

Widest part should be the largest measurement in this area

Widest measurement around the thighs

Widest measurement above the knees

Measurement record chart

DATE	WEIGHT	BUST	WAIST	HIPS	WIDEST PART

TOP OF THIGHS		ABOVE KNEES		UPPER ARMS		TOTAL INCHES/CM LOST THIS WEEK	TOTAL INCHES/CM LOST TO DATE
L	R	L	R	L	R		

Exercise planner

	M	T	W	T	F	S	S
Morning session							
Aerobic workout 30 minutes	☐	☐	☐	☐	☐	☐	☐
Toning exercises							
Hips and thighs	☐	☐	☐	☐	☐	☐	☐
Tummy and waist	☐	☐	☐	☐	☐	☐	☐
Lunchtime session							
Aerobic workout 30 minutes	☐	☐	☐	☐	☐	☐	☐
Toning exercises							
Hips and thighs	☐	☐	☐	☐	☐	☐	☐
Tummy and waist	☐	☐	☐	☐	☐	☐	☐
Afternoon/ evening session							
Aerobic workout 30 minutes	☐	☐	☐	☐	☐	☐	☐
Toning exercises							
Hips and thighs	☐	☐	☐	☐	☐	☐	☐
Tummy and waist	☐	☐	☐	☐	☐	☐	☐

Steps per day record chart

	DATE	TARGET STEPS	ACTUAL STEPS
Day 1			
Day 2			
Day 3			
Day 4			
Day 5			
Day 6			
Day 7			
Day 8			
Day 9			
Day 10			
Day 11			
Day 12			
Day 13			
Day 14			
Day 15			
Day 16			
Day 17			
Day 18			
Day 19			
Day 20			
Day 21			
Day 22			
Day 23			
Day 24			
Day 25			
Day 26			
Day 27			
Day 28			

Index of recipes

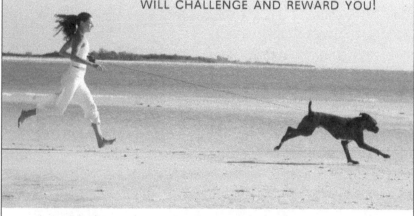
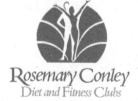
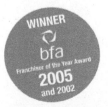

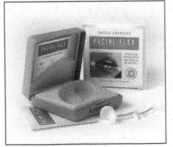
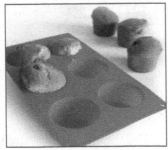
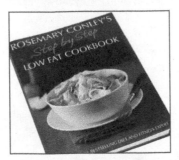
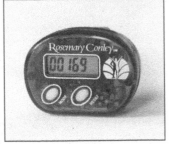
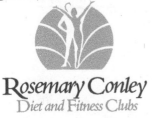

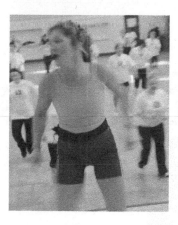
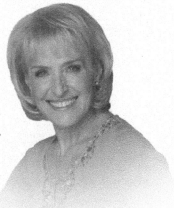

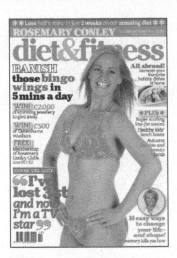

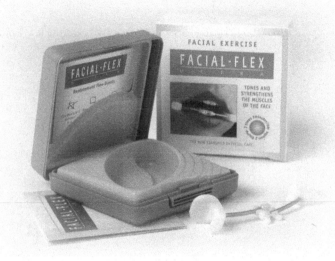
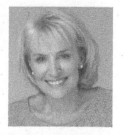

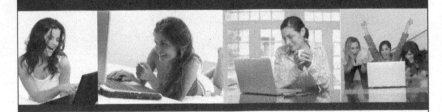
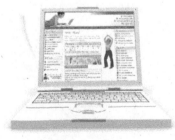